Examining Civic Engagement Links to Health

Findings from the Literature and
Implications for a Culture of Health

CHRISTOPHER NELSON, JENNIFER SLOAN, ANITA CHANDRA

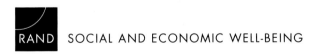

SOCIAL AND ECONOMIC WELL-BEING

Prepared for the Robert Wood Johnson Foundation

For more information on this publication, visit www.rand.org/t/RR3163

Library of Congress Cataloging-in-Publication Data is available for this publication.
ISBN: 978-1-9774-0344-5

Published by the RAND Corporation, Santa Monica, Calif.
© Copyright 2019 RAND Corporation
RAND® is a registered trademark.

Support RAND
Make a tax-deductible charitable contribution at
www.rand.org/giving/contribute

www.rand.org

Preface

The Robert Wood Johnson Foundation (RWJF) is leading a pioneering effort to advance a culture of health that "enables all members of our diverse society to lead healthier lives, now and for generations to come" (Plough, 2015). As noted in the Culture of Health Action Framework, achieving the goals of improved population health, well-being, and equity requires (1) changes in how people conceptualize, value, and engage around health issues (Action Area 1), (2) cross-sector partnerships to address the various social and economic determinants of health (Action Area 2), (3) communities that provide healthy environments in an equitable manner (Action Area 3), and (4) strengthened integration of health services and systems (Action Area 4) (Chandra, 2016).

Civic engagement (defined broadly as participating in activities that advance the public good) was identified as one of three drivers for Action Area 1, which focuses on ensuring that people value health and recognize the links between personal health decisions, community well-being investments, and community health outcomes. Like most aspects in a culture of health, the evidence base on civic engagement (e.g., voting, volunteering, social organizing, and other civic participation) is spread across various (mostly nonhealth) disciplines, is still mostly formative in terms of research rigor, and involves complex relationships among actors at the local, regional, national, and international levels. Furthermore, much of the empirical research comes from non-U.S. contexts—therefore, more study is needed on types of civic engagement and how that engagement operates within and across systems, cultures, and contexts. Additional in-depth analysis is needed to characterize and assess implications of what evidence does exist.

In this report, we conduct a structured review to understand what the scientific literature presents about the empirical relationship between health and civic engagement. We specifically examine whether health is a cause of civic engagement, a consequence of it, or both; what causal mechanisms underlie this link; and where there are gaps in knowledge for the field.

This report should be of interest to researchers and practitioners exploring the role of civic engagement in promoting health and well-being and identifying where investments and actions are needed. This report is intended to provide an initial overview on the published literature that examines associations between civic engagement and health outcomes. Future research should continue to unpack different approaches in civic engagement and how they vary by social and demographic context.

This research was sponsored by the Robert Wood Johnson Foundation and conducted within RAND Social and Economic Well-Being. Christopher Nelson led this research study. Questions about the report can be directed to cnelson@rand.org.

RAND Social and Economic Well-Being is a division of the RAND Corporation that seeks to actively improve the health and social and economic well-being of populations and communities throughout the world. This research was conducted in the Community Health and Environmental Policy Program within RAND Social and Economic Well-Being. The program focuses on such topics as infrastructure, science and technology, community design, community health promotion, migration and population dynamics, transportation, energy, and climate and the environment, as well as other policy concerns that are influenced by the natural and built environment, technology, and community organizations and institutions that affect well-being. For more information, email chep@rand.org.

Contents

Box, Figures, and Tables

Box

Figures

Tables

Summary

The Robert Wood Johnson Foundation (RWJF) is leading a pioneering effort to advance a culture of health that "enables all in our diverse society to lead healthier lives, now and for generations to come"(Plough, 2015). At the heart of the Culture of Health Action Framework are four action areas, the first of which is Making Health a Shared Value, which emphasizes the importance of achieving, maintaining, and reclaiming health as a shared priority. Civic engagement is one of the three drivers identified by RWJF for making progress in Action Area 1 (along with mindset and expectations, and sense of community). As noted by RWJF, through civic engagement, "people develop and use knowledge, skills and voice to cultivate positive change. Such actions can help improve the conditions that influence health and well-being for all. A civically engaged population demonstrates that people not only care about their community and nation but are also motivated to participate" (Robert Wood Johnson Foundation, undated).

Action Area 1 was informed by literature on health-related social movements.[1] This report seeks to build on and deepen those earlier analyses with a closer focus on the causal relationship between civic engagement and health and well-being—that is, whether better health and well-being might promote more civic engagement, whether civic engagement might promote health or well-being, or perhaps both. Specifically, we sought answers to the following questions:

---

[1] Anita Chandra, Carolyn E. Miller, Joie D. Acosta, Sarah Weilant, Matthew, Trujillo, and Alonzo Plough, "Drivers of Health as a Shared Value: Mindset, Expectations, Sense of Community, and Civic Engagement," *Health Affairs*, Vol. 35, No. 11, 2016, pp. 1959–1963.

- Is there an empirical relationship between health and/or well-being and civic engagement?
- Is health and/or well-being a cause of civic engagement, a consequence of it, or both?
- What causal mechanisms link civic engagement with health and/or well-being, and how can understanding the mechanisms influence programming or investment decisions?
- Is the nature of the health–civic engagement relationship different across various segments of the population?
- Where are the gaps in knowledge that might point to possible investment opportunities in new research?

This narrow focus is intended as a building block for additional reviews and analyses describing and characterizing the full range of interventions, social movements, and other efforts that use civic engagement as a tool for addressing the social determinants of health.

The analysis was based on English-language literature searches that identified articles with (1) a clear empirical measure of a health outcome, (2) a clear empirical measure of some aspect of civic engagement, and (3) evidence pertaining to the direction, size, and nature of the causal relationship between health and civic engagement. We defined *health* broadly to include physical health, mental health, and health-related behaviors. We define *well-being* in this context primarily as the subjective appraisal of life satisfaction and meaning. The definition of *civic engagement* is less precise in the literature but includes efforts by individuals and groups to influence laws, policies, regulations, and governmental practices that relate to health (Schlozman, Verba and Brady, 2012). This yielded a total of 1,329 results, from which two members of the team independently identified 157 articles for data abstraction, most of which were quantitative studies in peer-reviewed journals, and slightly more than half of which analyzed data from non-U.S. sources.

Is There an Empirical Relationship Between Health and Civic Engagement?

The majority of studies reviewed suggest that increases in physical and mental health and well-being are related to increases in civic engagement, whether through voting or through other activities, such as volunteering and membership in civic organizations. These findings held across a variety of health outcomes, including self-reported health, physical disability, mental health, the prevalence of healthy behaviors, and (in some cases) specific health conditions. Similarly, the health–civic engagement link applied to a variety of forms of civic engagement, including voting, membership in community organizations, volunteering, secular activism through churches, and others.

A few studies suggest that the effects of poor health on civic engagement are cumulative, both with multiple conditions (Sund et al., 2016) and with illnesses that last many years (Mattila et al., 2018). However, in many studies, the strength of the linkage varied in some cases among specific conditions; e.g., those with cancer sometimes were shown to be more prone to civic action than those with other conditions. In addition, there is evidence that the direction of the association varies across conditions—those with certain conditions were shown to have higher voting participation rates than those with other conditions (e.g., cancer versus asthma). Some authors speculate this may be related to differences in social stigma (e.g., the extent to which individuals are deemed responsible for their condition), sophistication of pressure groups formed around a condition, and more general differences in national culture.

Is Health a Cause of Civic Engagement, a Consequence of It, or Both?

The cross-sectional nature of most studies limits our ability to discern whether good health causes increases in civic engagement or vice versa. However, a small number of longitudinal studies suggest that poor health earlier in life is associated with lower levels of civic engagement later in life (Ojeda and Pacheco, 2017; Wray-Lake et al., 2017). Moreover, the effects seem to work in both directions—i.e., early depression is associated with less engagement later in life, and early civic engagement is associated with less depression later in life. There is evidence that the effects can persist for as long as 20 years (Pillemer et al., 2010).

What Causal Mechanisms Link Civic Engagement and Health?

Only a few studies we identified explicitly examine what causal mechanisms might link civic engagement and health. The most commonly referenced studies relate to the fact that poor health is often accompanied by increased social isolation, whether because of barriers to physical mobility or social stigma. This appears to hold for physical and mental health and such health-related behaviors as smoking. In addition, some studies suggest that the effects of civic engagement on health could be that of a buffer, lessening the negative effects on health of financial stress.

Is the Nature of the Health–Civic Engagement Relationship Different Across Different Segments of the Population?

A few studies make explicit comparisons among health conditions (e.g., cancer versus heart disease), but different studies arrived at different results about which conditions are associated with higher rates of civic engagement. There is also some evidence that the nature of the health–civic engagement connection may vary by racial group; for example, one study found that black cancer survivors were more likely to vote than white cancer survivors.

Where Are the Gaps in Knowledge That Might Point to Possible Investment Opportunities in New Research?

Although voting is a clearly defined activity, there appears to be less agreement about terminology and constructs for measuring civic engagement. This definitional discordance was present in the literature reviewed for this report. In addition, more research is needed that uses longitudinal designs to unpack causal relationships and further elucidates how health experience and voting behavior evolve over time. Furthermore, there is a relative dearth of studies seeking to link civic activism to broader concepts of well-being and just a few studies on civic engagement related to religious organizations. Perhaps most importantly, although there is a reasonable body of emerging evidence linking individual civic engagement to individual health, there is little attention to date on whether individual-level engagement is related to *community* health and conditions (e.g., infrastructure, policies) that shape health. This is key in understanding the extent to which civic engagement might fulfill its promise as a driver of improvements in health equity.

More research on how the driver of civic engagement operates across contexts is needed. For example, future work should unpack the role of different types of civic engagement (e.g., social and community organizing, grassroots advocacy, voting), how those civic engagement approaches vary by social and demographic context, and how effective strategies are in the context of crosscutting and systemic issues, such as health equity. Finally, much of the literature comes from non-U.S. contexts. Although there is a reasonably high degree of consistency in findings across countries, this material does raise questions about applicability to U.S.-based funders and decisionmakers.

Given this initial analysis, the following are next steps that RWJF and other funders might consider:

- **Improve availability and analysis of robust longitudinal and multilevel data sets.** Research in this area requires merging data sets on health with those on voting and other forms of civic engagement, which creates an extra hurdle for researchers.

Funders should consider supporting the creation, maintenance, and analysis of thorough, longitudinal data sets to further understand the mechanisms underlying the health–civic engagement link.

- **Support research that specifically targets causal mechanisms.** Although several studies suggest that the health–civic engagement link is found in the role that poor health plays in increasing social isolation, more research is needed to deepen our understanding of this and to explore other possible mechanisms.

- **Support research that examines how civic engagement influences structural and systemic barriers to health.** Although this study was limited to the linkages between civic engagement and health, additional work is needed to explore the connections between civic engagement and the various social determinants of health, along with pathways through which civic engagement changes equity-based policies and environments and community power structures in ways that shape health.

- **Support the development and sustainment of multidisciplinary communities of practice.** Work in this area involves an ability to blend expertise and perspectives from public health and from political science, sociology and other social/behavior sciences. Funders should consider sponsoring conferences, forums, and networks to provide venues in which researchers can collaborate (specifically around shared data sets, as mentioned above) and more actively contribute articles to build the literature base.

- **Support collaborative intervention design within communities of practice.** Sound intervention design requires knowledge of potential causal mechanisms that might be leveraged, practical knowledge of how to design and implement cost-effective, feasible interventions, and the evaluation capacity needed to systematically track implementation and assess causality. Support for forums involving individuals and organizations with these various skill sets may help speed up the process of identifying ways to both promote civic engagement and realize any related health benefits.

- **Support investigation into how health-related civic engagement relates to other forms of engagement.** More work is needed to understand the mechanisms underlying community organizing, advocacy, social mobilization, and other forms of participation and the relative effects on health outcomes.

Acknowledgments

We appreciate the guidance and input received in the review of this report by Amanda Navarro of PolicyLink and Malcolm Williams of the RAND Corporation. We are also thankful for the expert assistance of project librarian Jody Larkin in conducting the searches and accessing the articles, Serafina Lana for expert research assistance, and Laura Coley for editorial and other assistance. We also thank Aditi Vaidya, Carolyn Miller, and Matthew Trujillo of the Robert Wood Johnson Foundation for their vision and support of this work.

Abbreviations

CBO	community-based organization
CMD	Common Mental Disorder
EYA	early young adulthood
FLTI	Family Leadership Training Institute
RWJF	Robert Wood Johnson Foundation

CHAPTER ONE

Background

The Robert Wood Johnson Foundation (RWJF) is leading a pioneering effort to advance a culture of health that "enables all in our diverse society to lead healthier lives, now and for generations to come" (Plough, 2015). As noted in the Culture of Health Action Framework (see Figure 1.1), achieving the goals of improved population health, well-being, and equity requires (1) changes in how people conceptualize, value, and engage around health issues (Action Area 1), (2) cross-sector partnerships to address the various social and economic determinants of health (Action Area 2), (3) communities that provide healthy environments in an equitable manner (Action Area 3), and (4) strengthened integration of health services and systems (Action Area 4) (Chandra et al., 2016).

Action Area 1 (Making Health a Shared Value) is where the cultural change aspects of the Culture of Health Action Framework is most evident. Action Area 1 emphasizes the importance of achieving, maintaining, and reclaiming health as a shared priority. RWJF identified three drivers of change needed to make progress in this Action Area: (1) mindset and expectations (how the U.S. public views and prioritizes health, well-being, and related investments); (2) sense of community (whether and how people feel connected to their communities, and how that connection can foster shared health values); and (3) civic engagement (interest in promoting or advocating for health and well-being topics for self and others). As noted by RWJF, through civic engagement, "people develop and use knowledge, skills and voice to cultivate positive change. Such actions can help improve the con-

Figure 1.1
Culture of Health Action Framework

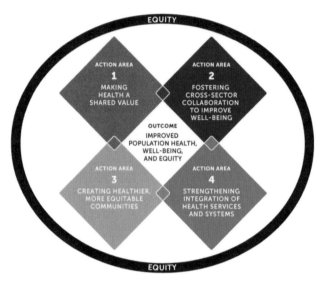

SOURCE: Robert Wood Johnson Foundation

ditions that influence health and well-being for all. A civically engaged population demonstrates that people not only care about their community and nation but are also motivated to participate" (Robert Wood Johnson Foundation, undated).

Making Health a Shared Value draws on research regarding how communities develop shared values for social priorities and the primary mechanisms involved in creating those shared values (see Box 1 for more information on the drivers related to Action Area 1). Among the most-notable findings from the research informing this Action Area is that values are the "major link between culture and action" (Cornish et al., 2014). Moreover, large-scale social change in other areas, such as environmental sustainability or tobacco use, has come from shifts in mindset and changes in the priorities of key actors (Brown and Fee, 2014). In health-related social movements (i.e., social movements to facilitate an improvement in a specific health outcome), however, the current focus is primarily on disease recognition and less on more-holistic notions of health, well-being, and equity. Thus, there is

Box 1: Examples of Research Basis for Action Area 1 Drivers

- **Mindset and expectations.** The fields of sociology and anthropology note that "social change requires collective action through movement in perspective, shared narrative, and cultural meaning" (Chandra et al., 2016)—in other words, this action requires a change in mindset among other cultural shifts. A mindset shift in health is currently most evident in single intervention and single health issue causes (e.g., tobacco control) (Siegal, Siegal, and Bonnie, 2009; Merzel and D'Afflitti, 2003).

- **Sense of community.** Previous research shows that individuals who live in places with a strong sense of community are healthier, and that sense of community contributes to greater civic participation and group-based belief systems that can promote shared values (Davidson and Cotter, 1991; Wu and Chow, 2013)

- **Civic engagement.** Civic engagement signals investment in community and has been linked to better outcomes in adulthood (Ballard, Hoyt, and Pachucki, 2019). Some studies are emerging now on the value of citizen engaged research/citizen science in monitoring community health outcomes (Den Broeder et al., 2018).

need for more analysis on the *mechanisms* through which a community mindset can be developed for health broadly, and how these shifts in views facilitate greater civic engagement for health overall.

This report seeks to contribute to the development of the knowledge base surrounding Action Area 1 by summarizing and exploring the implications of existing evidence on the third driver—civic engagement (specifically on the link between civic engagement and health/well-being). This initial review focuses on the question of whether there is evidence that civic engagement is causally related to health—that is, whether better health promotes more civic engagement, whether civic engagement promotes health, or perhaps both. Specifically, we sought to ascertain what existing scientific literature suggests about the following questions:

- Is there an empirical relationship between health and civic engagement?
- Is health a cause of civic engagement, a consequence of it, or both ?
- What causal mechanisms link civic engagement and health, and how can understanding the mechanisms influence programming or investment decisions?
- Is the nature of the health–civic engagement relationship different across different segments of the population?
- Where are the gaps in knowledge that might point to possible investment opportunities in new research?

Chapter Two of this report describes the scope of the review and methods used for it. The chapters following summarize findings related to (1) voting and (2) other forms of civic engagement, such as volunteering and membership in civic organizations. The rationale for treating voting separately is that, in democratic systems, voting provides a regular opportunity to influence not just specific health conditions and communities (through state, regional, and national elections) but also the identities and preferences of those making policies related to health and the full range of other collective issues. We note that there are more forms of civic engagement than are summarized in this report, such as community organizing and advocacy. However, the majority of the studies in current peer-reviewed journals focus on usual or more-formal forms of civic engagement as directly linked to traditional health outcomes. This report concludes by summarizing what existing literature says about each of the questions above and by identifying some possible next steps for RWJF and other funders.

Before proceeding, we offer one note about the scope of this research. Reviewing literature describing and characterizing the full range of interventions, social movements, and other efforts that use civic engagement as a tool for addressing the social determinants of health was beyond the scope of this initial study. These elements also are key to Action Area 1 (Making Health a Shared Value). Therefore, more formal study and rigorous research of how the driver of civic engagement operates across contexts is needed. For example, future work should unpack the role of different types of civic engagement (e.g., social and community organizing, grassroots advocacy, voting), how those civic engagement approaches vary by social and demographic context, and how effective strategies are in the context of crosscutting and systemic issues, such as health equity.

CHAPTER TWO

Methods

Scoping the review required making decisions about how to conceptualize *health* and *civic engagement*, both of which are open to multiple interpretations. In keeping with the *culture of health* definition and Culture of Health Action Framework, we define *health* broadly to include physical health, mental health, and health-related behaviors. We also include both individual- and community-level health outcomes, as well as the concept of well-being. It should be noted that there are upstream drivers of health (e.g., social, political, and economic drivers) that can also be considered secondary or concurrent health outcomes and are certainly central to health equity. However, for the purposes of this report, we needed to focus first on more proximal health outcomes.

Defining *civic engagement* is a bit more challenging. In democratic systems like the United States, voting is the most common and widespread way in which individuals can influence laws, policies, regulations, and governmental practices that relate to health (Schlozman, Verba, and Brady, 2012). However, health is also affected by many factors outside the scope of government and public policy. Thus, we also examined other aspects of civic engagement, such as volunteerism, membership in civic organizations, and attending civic or community meetings. However, we omitted literature on political activities (e.g., lobbying, campaign contributions) by health-related professional organizations and unions (e.g., the American Medical Association, nurse's unions) for the purposes of this review because we were principally focused on the motivations of individuals.

With these general definitions in mind, we used the Scopus data-base to run English-language searches on "civic engagement," "civic action," "(voter OR voting) AND (registration OR turnout OR partici-pation)," "community advocacy," "community organizing," and "civic participation." Scopus was selected because it captures a broader disci-plinary base of articles from health sciences, political science, and other social sciences. Each term was paired with "health" and "well-being." This yielded a total of 1,329 results, from which two members of the team independently identified 157 articles for data abstraction, most of which were quantitative studies in peer-reviewed journals. Although we included such terms as "community organizing" or "advocacy" in our search, it is entirely possible that there is research not represented in these databases that would capture the health effects of less formal civic engagement.

We conducted an abstract review of 157 studies (see Figure 2.1). Of those, we determined that 109 were relevant and the full report should be reviewed, and 48 were not relevant because they did not report on a civic engagement–related outcome or a health or well-being outcome. Of the 109 articles that were reviewed in full, we included 64 research studies in this report, and ten additional studies evaluating civic engagement interventions. Articles were included in this report

Figure 2.1
Literature Search Process

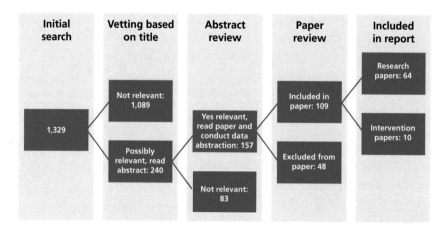

only if they included (1) a clear empirical measure of a health outcome, (2) a clear empirical measure of some aspect of civic engagement, and (3) evidence pertaining to the direction, size, and nature of the causal relationship between health and civic engagement. We also included a small number of qualitative studies that included an explicit attempt to characterize or explore specific causal mechanisms linking health and civic engagement. However, our inclusion criteria imply that our analysis does not fully reflect the range of more ethnographic studies, which can illuminate causal relationships but in less direct ways. We also did not capture the full range of articles describing interventions involving the civic engagement-health nexus, except those that were part of structured or empirically based evaluations that met the conditions stated above.

Many of the studies that we located are based on data collected outside the United States, mostly notably in Europe and the Scandinavian countries. We included these studies in large part because of the modest number of U.S.-based studies. In addition, we judged that it would be better to treat U.S.–versus–non-U.S. differences in the health–civic engagement link as an empirical question rather than excluding studies based on assumptions about cross-national differences. We recognize that there are limitations in some aspects of transferability across diverse political and demographic contexts, but it is important to surface information about the links between civic engagement and health outcomes in the most rigorous studies available to date.

During our title vetting, articles were included in the "possibly relevant" bucket if there was any indication that they might relate to civic engagement, health, and well-being. Articles deemed not relevant based on title were articles that were very clearly not relevant to these keywords, such as articles focused on computer ethics, waterborne illnesses, or companion animals. In the abstract review, articles were deemed "relevant" if there was any mention of health or well-being and civic engagement (e.g., engagement in social organizations, civic organizations, volunteering), voting, or the related area of social capital. All countries, populations, measurement tools, and study designs were accepted into the article review round, including overview articles and commentaries, as long as relevance was apparent. In the article review, we excluded articles that, after a closer look, did not reflect health or well-being or any type of civic engagement, or examined the overall health of democracy, not human health outcomes. A complete list of all articles included in the review is provided in Appendix B, and a more detailed table with key study findings and attributes is provided in Appendix C.

Articles selected for final review were coded using a data abstraction form (see Appendix A) that noted the region or country of the study, the subpopulation of interest, the year(s) that data were collected, how civic engagement was measured, what health outcomes were included and how they were measured, sample size and sample description, and key findings. Given the exploratory intent of the review, we took a broad view on what types of studies might provide evidence pertaining to the causal link between health and civic engagement. Only one study (noted below) used randomized control designs because of the impracticality of randomly assigning individuals to different health or civic engagement conditions. Thus, we also assigned articles into three groups based on the methods used to assess empirical relationships and causality: (1) longitudinal quantitative studies that afford the opportunity to explore temporal sequences of events, (2) cross-sectional quantitative studies with statistical controls, and (3) qualitative and descriptive studies that included a clear attempt to document and explore causal mechanisms linking health and civic engagement. Given the multiplicity of outcome measures used, we made no attempt to quantitatively compile the strength of findings. In light of the study's exploratory intent, we set no minimum quality standards for inclusion into the study (other than peer review) and chose instead to present a sensitivity analysis (see Chapter Six) exploring whether the nature of the conclusions differed across quality ratings.

CHAPTER THREE

Health and Voting Participation

We begin with key findings from studies related to voting participation and health. Most of these studies focus not on whether voters lean toward one party, ideology, or candidate, but on whether they vote at all. However, we do note that two studies link health to preferences for parties or candidates.

Studies of voting and other forms of democratic participation have been a staple of political science, political sociology, and political psychology since the end of World War II, when scientists took advantage of newly emerging approaches to surveys and sampling to understand the workings of democratic systems and transitions to democracy in the post-colonial era. This vast literature includes various approaches focusing on individual decisionmaking (Downs, 1957; Bobo and Gilliam, 1990) and resources (Verba and Nie, 1972), social groupings (Hobbs, Christakis, and Fowler, 2014), and such institutional features as voting registration procedures (Highton, 2017).

Health, however, has received relatively little attention as a potential driver of voter participation. As Gollust and Rahn (2015) note, given that we know health and healthy behaviors and environments are not equitably distributed, if there is a connection to voting and if voting affects policy influencing health (Goetzel et al., 2003; Navarro and Shi, 2001), then this could result in an amplifying mechanism for inequity. Furthermore, if the causal relationship runs the other way and voting improves health, this could result in a cycle in which those who start out with strong health and good civic habits do get progressively better, while others get progressively worse (Wolstenholme, 2003). We emphasize that the evidence base does *not* yet support such conclusions, but we raise these possibilities to underscore the importance of this topic.

In the remainder of this chapter, we consider the relationship between the propensity to vote and physical health, behavioral, and mental health. Although most of the evidence relates to the health of *individuals*, we describe a small number of studies on *community-level* health at the end of the chapter.

Voting and Physical Health

Several studies explore the relationship between physical health and the propensity to vote. Some studies examine general health, while others focus on specific aspects of health.

Voting and Self-Rated Health

We begin with seven studies of self-rated health, a commonly used indicator of general health. Various large-sample survey studies from Europe during the 2000s provide evidence that those who report lower levels of health are less likely to vote in elections. For example, an analysis of responses from the National Child Development Study, a longitudinal study of all people living in Ireland and Britain who were born in one week in March 1958 examined correlates of voting in the 1979, 1987, and 1997 elections (sample sizes were 8,463, 6,653, and 6,782, respectively), and found that individuals with poor self-rated health were significantly less likely to report voting in past general elections (Denny and Doyle, 2007). Some authors speculate that poor health might weaken an individual's social network (Mattila et al., 2013). In one of the most recent and high-quality studies, Mattila et al. (2013) analyzed data from more than 200,000 respondents across 30 European countries in the 2002, 2004, 2006, 2008, and 2010 European Social Surveys, finding that self-reported general health ("very good," "good," "fair," "bad," or "very bad") was related to turnout and was partly mediated by social connectedness. The authors suggested that attenuated health might weaken an individual's social network, which in turn depresses voting. That is, people who participate in social activities and meet with friends, colleagues, or relatives have a higher propensity to vote than people with more-restricted social relations. Thus, when social activity is controlled for, the effect of health is discernibly attenuated, which supports the interpretation that health has also an indirect effect on turnout.

A research team from Ireland (Kelleher et al., 2002) conducted a study of data on 6,539 voters from 18 of 273 representative district electoral divisions in Ireland's 1997 elections. They examined the cross-sectional relationship between mortality patterns, indicators of deprivation, general lifestyle, and social attitudes, as exemplified by general election voting patterns. The authors found that various measures of social deprivation (including lower rates of voting) were related to lower levels of health.[1] Because it is based on a series of bivariate correlations, the design of this study limits the conclusions that can be drawn about causality.

Another study used a government data set of 2009 national election voter turnout in Denmark (i.e., not just self-reported voting). Bhatti and Hansen (2012) found that voter turnout among 90-year-olds in Denmark was 30 percentage points less than among 60-year-olds. Lower levels of health among the 90-year-olds (measured by the number of times a respondent was admitted to a hospital and days spent in the hospital) explained some of the difference. But the authors speculated that much of the decline could be explained by the disruption of social ties accompanied with withdrawing from the labor market and a greater tendency to live alone. Voter turnout declines faster for women than it does for men. The authors speculate that this could be because women lose their social network earlier than men, because they are, on average, widowed and live alone at an earlier age than men, and because women live longer and are typically younger than their husbands. Also, older

---

[1]   This is also one a few studies we located that explored the relationship between health and voter preference among candidates and parties. These studies also found that left-wing voting associated with increased mortality, but the relationship was neither strong nor clear (which they attribute to the fact that the two major parties were both center-right during that time).

generations of women are also less educated and have lower job market affiliation than men.

Another study focused on disabilities, linking disability to a lower propensity to vote. Analyzing cross-sectional data from a nationally representative random-household telephone survey in 1998 of 1,240 U.S. adults (with oversampling for disabled adults), Schur et al. (2002) found that people with disabilities were 20 percentage points less likely to vote in the 1998 midterm election than people without disabilities who had similar demographic characteristics. The researchers found that other standard predictors (e.g., sense of efficacy, being contacted by parties) explained only a small fraction of this gap. To illustrate the magnitude of the participation gap, the authors calculated that if individuals who had disabilities voted at the same rate as those without disabilities, there would have been about 4.6 million more voters in 1998, raising the overall turnout rate by 2.4 percentage points.

Although the cross-sectional nature of the aforementioned studies limits efforts to assess the direction of causality, a study of 9,000 youths from the National Longitudinal Study of Youth analyzed the relationship between levels and trajectories in self-reported health (e.g., chronic physical conditions, mental health) and levels and trajectories in voter turnout in the 2004 and 2008 U.S. presidential elections and the 2006 and 2010 midterm elections (Ojeda and Pacheco, 2017). The authors found that certain conditions dampen the probability of voting in spite of changes in young adulthood, such as education, mobilization, and familiarization with the political process that typically leads to a positive voting trajectory during this period. Specifically, (1) lower self-rated health reduced the initial probability of voting but not the slope (i.e., rate of increase) of the voting trajectory; (2) depression slowed (and sometimes even reversed) an individual's voting trajectory; and (3) physical limitations did not have a statistically significant effect on either the initial probability of voting or a citizen's trajectory in young adulthood—however, the authors do not rule out the possibility of an effect later in life.

Finally, one study provides an explicit comparison of the effects of poor health on voting with other forms of civic participation. Söderlund and Rapeli (2015) analyzed a 2012–2013 cross section of more than

8,000 respondents to the European Social Survey data for Denmark, Finland, Iceland, Norway, and Sweden. The authors explored the links between self-reported health ("very good," "good," and "fair/bad/very bad") and political participation, such as voting; work in a political party or action group; displaying a campaign badge or sticker; contacting a politician, government or local government official; taking part in a lawful public demonstration; signing a petition; and boycotting certain products. Like the studies mentioned above, researchers found that respondents reporting good health were more likely to vote than those with poor health. However, this group found what they termed a "reverse health gap" with other forms of political participation. Specifically, respondents with poor health were more active than their healthy counterparts in direct contacts with power holders (i.e., reaching out to political leaders directly), participation in demonstrations, and wearing a campaign button. The findings might suggest that, under some conditions, poor health can stimulate people into other forms of political engagement, such as attending a rally. One possible explanation of the reverse health gap might relate to differences in the characteristics of various health conditions, which is addressed in the next set of studies we examined.

Voting and Other Physical Health Conditions

Four articles in this review focus on indicators of morbidity and mortality, or on specific conditions (such as cancer or influenza), often finding different voting results for different health conditions. For example, Sund et al. (2016) combined an individual-level, registry-based data set that contained an 11-percent random sample of the entire electorate in the 1999 Finnish parliamentary elections. This data set had information on hospital discharge diagnoses and reimbursements for drugs prescribed. Conducting a cross-sectional analysis, after adjusting for gender, age, education, occupational class, income, partnership status, cohabitation with underaged children, and hospitalization during Election Day, the authors found that although alcoholism and mental disorders had a negative association with voting, cancer, chronic obstructive pulmonary disorder (COPD), and/or asthma had a positive association (both odds ratios = 1.05) with voting.

Gollust and Rahn (2015) analyzed cross-sectional data from eight states (49,405 respondents) from the 2009 Behavioral Risk Factor Surveillance Survey to examine the associations between having diagnoses of five chronic conditions and turnout in the 2008 U.S. presidential election. After adjusting for sociodemographic characteristics and some health-related confounding factors, they found that individuals with cancer diagnoses are more likely to vote, while those with heart disease diagnoses are less likely to vote. These associations differed by race and educational status; notably, blacks and those with lower education who also had cancer were more likely to vote than whites and those with more education who also had cancer. The authors noted that the differences in the health-to-voting relationship for cancer versus heart disease could be related to a social stigma associated with cultural perceptions that heart disease, unlike cancer, is a result of poor individual behavior and choices. The researchers cited evidence that cancer patients are more likely to self-identify as "survivors," which is more empowering than "victim." They also provided descriptive evidence that there are better-organized groups mobilized around cancer than there are around heart disease, and these groups might help to encourage voting.

Finally, we identified two studies that examined the effects of multiple health conditions on the propensity to vote. The aforementioned report by Sund et al. (2016) found that having more than one condition at a time further decreased voting probability. Similarly, a large-sample study (which included analysis of official records for 204,034 randomly selected individuals in Finland who were eligible to vote in the 1999 parliamentary elections, 16,170 who were eligible for the 2012 presidential elections, and 32,768 for the 2012 municipal elections) found that multiple illnesses over *several* years were more strongly connected to decreases in turnout than health problems experienced only in the year before the elections (Mattila et al., 2018). Falling ill at the time of the elections had no consistent additional negative relationship with voting. The authors speculated that long-term effects on voting are related to lower levels of political efficacy, interest, and social connectedness.

Although not directly in the scope of the analysis, it is interesting to note that the health-voting nexus also appears to relate to access to health care, which could partially reflect perceived poor health and also something that conceivably could be a separate driver for people to act politically. Ziegenfuss, Davern, and Blewett (2008) showed (using a retrospective, pre-post design) that a higher proportion of participants in the American National Election Study reported difficulty in 2004 regarding access to health care than in 2000, that a larger share of those reporting such difficulties voted in 2004 than in 2000, and that their preferences shifted to more heavily favor the Democratic candidate.

Voting and Behavioral and Mental Health

Some studies focus specifically on the health-voting connection in the context of behavioral and mental health. The next sections summarize those findings, starting with behavioral choices.

Voting and Health Behaviors

There are three studies in this review that link health behaviors, such as smoking and drinking, with voting. In an analysis of 11,626 respondents in Colorado's 2005–2006 Tobacco Attitudes and Behaviors Survey, those who reported smoking were less than half as likely to vote in the 2004 election as those who did not (Albright et al., 2015). The Colorado study's authors suggested that the findings might relate to earlier Swedish findings that smokers are marginalized, less likely to have trust in institutions, less inclined to participate politically, and that continuing to smoke is related to lack of social networks (Lindström, 2009). Although the study did not directly point to mechanisms, the authors in the Swedish study suggested two options: (1) that the stigma associated with smoking might motivate some to quit but might cause others to withdraw from social networks, and (2) that efforts in the political arena to limit smoking (e.g., through higher taxation) lead smokers to feel aggrieved and alienated from the political system.

Denny and Doyle (2007) found that British smokers were 4 percent less likely than nonsmokers to vote in the 1979 and 1997 elections and 3 percent less likely to vote in the 1987 election. Interestingly, moderate drinkers were *more* likely to report voting in the two previous elections than nondrinkers, while heavy drinkers were more likely to report voting in the 1997 election, something the authors speculate might be related to the social nature of drinking and pub culture. If true, this hypothesis might support other studies suggesting that health affects voting in part through social isolation (a finding that might not hold in the United States, which does not have the long-standing pub culture that is found in the United Kingdom [UK]).

Another perspective on the relationship between voting and health behaviors comes from a study by Mino et al. (2011), which assessed the relationship of risk reduction, substance use, and voting. The study focused on a cross section of 162 individuals recruited at six New York City methadone clinics participating in HIV programs between 2005 and 2007. The team surveyed respondents on various measures of political engagement (e.g., being registered to vote, following politics, identifying with a political party) and found these measures were associated with a higher prevalence of healthy behaviors, such as a lower likelihood of needle-sharing and lower use of injection shooting galleries. This suggests that maintaining connections with mainstream civic activities can be related to individuals taking precautions to reduce health risks, including HIV risk. This is important in a population that could be considered less healthy and marginalized and perhaps less likely to engage given prior study findings on poor self-reported health and lower voting.

Voting and Mental Health

There are nine studies in this review that focus on voting and mental health. Four of those focus on voting and depression specifically. Ojeda (2015) examined the effects of depression on voter participation using data from a large-sample, three-wave study covering 1994–1995, 1995–

1996, and 2001–2002.[2] The study used data from the General Social Survey and the National Longitudinal Study of Adolescent Health to follow individuals from middle and high school into adulthood. The analysis found that both adult and adolescent depression reduced the probability of political participation, an effect that holds even after controlling for age and education (primary predictors of turnout); key demographic characteristics, such as race, gender, and class; and a host of plausible confounding factors, such as partisan strength, general health, church attendance, and happiness. The author speculates that the linkage could be related to sleep problems and feelings of hopelessness and apathy.

Additional longitudinal studies demonstrate that depressive symptoms early in life may decrease later voting. One large, U.S.-based study suggested that adolescent and early young adulthood depressive symptoms predicted decreases in later voting, and community engagement in the same groups predicted decreases in later depressive symptoms (Wray-Lake et al., 2017). The researchers provided preliminary evidence on this trajectory through analysis of 15,701 observations from the 1995, 2001, and 2008 iterations of the National Longitudinal Study of Adolescent Health. The authors examined the directional relationship between various forms of social and civic engagement (e.g., extracurricular engagement, involvement in service and organizations, time spent volunteering or on community service activities) and depression (e.g., "Did you vote and are you registered to vote?" "How often you are likely to vote in local/state elections?" "High-cost political actions: contributing money to a party or candidate, contacting a representative, participating in political orgs, attending a political rally/march"). Results of longitudinal, structural equation models suggested that adolescent and early young adulthood (EYA) depressive symptoms predicted decreases in later voting. Adolescent and EYA community engagement predicted decreases in later depressive symptoms. Analyses suggested that findings held across gender, age, socioeconomic status, race/ethnicity, and EYA social roles. The results demonstrated that

---

[2] Wave 1 included 20,745 respondents, wave 2 had 14,738 respondents, and wave 3 had 15,197 respondents.

community engagement might have mental health benefits for youths, and that depression might reduce later civic engagement in adulthood.

In another study (also discussed earlier in the "Voting and Self-Rated Health" subsection of this chapter), analysis of responses from 9,000 U.S. youths examined the relationship between levels or trajectories in self-reported health and voter turnout. The authors found that depression dampens the likelihood of voting in spite of other life-course factors that could otherwise facilitate voting engagement (e.g., increasing education, familiarization with the political process, etc.) as people mature (Ojeda and Pacheco, 2017). Similarly, the aforementioned Finnish study by Sund et al. (2016) found that—after adjusting for gender, age, education, occupational class, income, partnership status, cohabitation with underaged children, and hospitalization during Election Day—mental disorders also had a negative association with voting.

The previously mentioned study by Denny and Doyle (2007) found a negative relationship between turnout in the 1987 election and mental health, measured using the malaise inventory scale, a self-report survey of psychological and somatic symptoms; however, this effect was negligible and statistically significant only in the 1987 sample.

Other studies examine the relationship between mental health and voting among individuals in inpatient and outpatient settings. Although these samples examine specific populations of interest and are thus less generalizable to the general population, they provide an opportunity to examine those at most risk of exclusion from political life because of health conditions. For example, a survey of 100 outpatients with dementia during the two months following the November 2000 U.S. presidential election (Ott, Heindel and Papandonatos, 2003) found that although a majority (60 percent) voted, increasing severity of dementia was associated with reduced knowledge about the election as well as reduced voting participation by patients—and also by caregivers. Actively voting people had general knowledge about the election as evidenced by matching candidate photographs with name and party labels.

Similarly, in an overview of the literature, Kelly (2014) examined the voting rates of psychiatry inpatients in Ireland, Germany, Israel, and Canada. The voting rate of psychiatric inpatients is much lower than the national rate and sometimes as low as 3 percent, despite evidence that psychiatric inpatients are well-informed voters and that a majority of those who do vote report feelings of responsibility, belonging to their community, and pride (Kelly, 2014). The literature demonstrates that the low voting rate among psychiatry inpatients and individuals with mental illness might be the result of issues of access, administrative issues (e.g., lack of an identity card), lack of knowledge, and neglect from political candidates because of a perception that individuals with mental illness do not vote.

Bosquet et al. (2009) conducted an observational study of all French inpatients of an internal medicine department in a hospital just outside Paris during the French presidential and legislative elections in 2007. The objectives of the study were to determine turnout among all registered inpatients and to assess the voting experience, reasons for abstention, medical and cognitive ability of voters, and how voting related to the Mini-Mental State Examination score. Of the 81 participants who were eligible to participate in the study and who were registered to vote, only 22 voted in the election (21 by proxy and one in person). The primary reasons that inpatients chose not to vote were: medical reasons ($n = 8$), personal reasons ($n = 8$), and the way the hospital organized the voting procedures ($n = 22$). The authors also stressed the importance of assessing the cognitive ability of voters, especially where proxy voting is concerned. They noted that hospital staff often function as gatekeepers to the voting process and make assumptions based on how they perceived patient mental competence, which could have resulted in some patients' exclusion from voting.

Another study focused on patients seeking mental health services. Kelly and Nash (2018) conducted a descriptive analysis of data from a cross-sectional survey of 117 participants in Irish mental health services (30 of whom were inpatients) after the 2016 general election, finding that although 82 percent were registered to vote, only 52 percent actually voted. Inpatients (20 percent) were substantially less likely to vote than outpatients (63 percent). Forty-one percent reported having insufficient information about voting: the most common information deficits related to voting rights (31.6 percent) and voting in hospital

(18.8 percent). The most common reasons for not voting were being in hospital (32.1 percent) and not being registered (30.4 percent).

Voting and Community Health

Although the majority of studies we located examine the health-voting linkage at the individual level, three studies provided evidence of such a linkage at the *community* level. First, a pair of studies examined the linkage between community-level voting participation rates and influenza prevalence. An analysis of district and regional voter turnout in the United States and Finland (1995–2015) found that influenza outbreaks were associated with lower voting rates (Blakely, Kennedy, and Kawachi, 2001; Urbatsch, 2017). Urbatsch (2017) examined the relationship between regional turnout rates in Finland (district level) and the United States (state level) from 1995 to 2015 with measures of local influenza prevalence. In both countries, regression models suggested that influenza outbreaks were associated with lower voting rates. This provides some evidence that the individual-level linkages between health and civic engagement could also apply to the broader community level. The remaining studies involving community health involve outcomes other than voter turnout but are included for consideration. Turning from acute to chronic conditions, another study examined the linkage between community obesity rates and voter candidate preference. Shin and McCarthy (2013), focusing at the county rather than individual level, found that higher 2009 age-adjusted obesity prevalence (with a BMI greater than 30) was associated with stronger support for U.S. presidential candidate Mitt Romney in 2012. Based on an analysis of party platforms, the authors used candidate preference as a proxy for how voters viewed solutions to the obesity problem: personal responsibility versus "government sponsored, multi-sectoral efforts."[3]

---

[3]   Specifically, the authors note that the 2012 Republican platform stated, "When approximately 80% of healthcare costs are related to lifestyle—smoking, obesity, substance abuse—far greater emphasis has to be put upon personal responsibility for health maintenance," which echoed their 2008 platform that noted, "We can reduce demand for medical care by

The implication, accordingly to the study authors, is that a large number of obese voters endorsed the personal-responsibility frame.

In one of the few studies to explicitly address equity issues, Blakely, Kennedy, and Kawachi (2001) analyzed pooled cross sections of a multilevel sample of 279,066 respondents to the 1990, 1992, 1994, and 1996 Current Population Survey, finding that individuals living in the states with the highest voting inequality (using an index created by the authors that used state-level inequality in voting turnout by family income and educational attainment) had 43 percent greater odds of rating their health as fair or poor than individuals living in the states with the lowest voting inequality. Although the authors found no direct association between voting and income inequality, when voting and income inequality are combined into one measure of inequality, people living in the nine most unequal states had 54 percent greater odds of fair or poor self-rated health than people living in the 19 most egalitarian states. The authors speculated (based on other literature) that the reasons for the voting inequality-health connection might include (1) adverse physiological consequences of being lower in the socioeconomic hierarchy and (2), relatedly, that increased inequality amplifies psychosocial comparisons up and down the hierarchy. This suggests that socioeconomic inequality in voter turnout is associated with poor self-rated health, independent of both income inequality and state median household income. Interestingly, the inequality-health linkage was smaller among blacks, although the authors provide no explanation of why this might be the case.

Summary

Although the research on voting and health would benefit from further development, particularly in the United States, the studies to date demonstrate some important associations. At the individual level, poor self-reported health is associated with lower voting participation rates.

---

fostering personal responsibility within a culture of wellness" (Republican National Committee, 2012; Republican National Committee, 2008).

With the exception of some specific chronic diseases (e.g., cancer versus asthma), most research shows that the burden of chronic disease also is related to less engagement in voting behaviors. Similarly, engagement in unhealthy behaviors (e.g., substance use) and experience of depression appears negatively correlated with voting participation. The mechanisms for this association between poor health and voting appears to be related to difficulty participating in activities given health burden, social isolation or marginalization from having a health concern, and a lack of trust in institutions that might be fostered or exacerbated by poor health status. Additional investigation into the role of these structural and systemic barriers in driving health and voting behavior (simultaneously or in concert) might inform the development of interventions seeking to augment civic engagement by more historically underrepresented populations.

CHAPTER FOUR

Other Forms of Civic Engagement

We turn next to studies that examine other forms of civic engagement, which we define as efforts to use voluntary collective action to address an issue of public or collective concern. Although Chapter Three focused on voting, this chapter addresses all other forms of civic engagement addressed in the articles generated by the literature search. Specific examples include organizational membership, participation, and volunteering. In cases for which the potential effects of such engagement activities can be limited—i.e., to specific communities, neighborhoods, or even individuals—the effects are often more directly linked to the efforts of specific individuals. Moreover, election of favored candidates is no guarantee that they will be able to pass laws, and passage of laws is no guarantee that they will be implemented and have an effect. Therefore, these engagement activities, although often more limited in scope or reach, are potential important vehicles of change.

In many instances, civic engagement is conceptualized as part of the broader construct of social capital. However, we include only those studies that contained a clear and specific measure of civic engagement as a part of the broader social capital construct. Furthermore, we included articles on membership in churches and religious organizations only when there was clear evidence that such membership entails civic activism (i.e., more than prayer or introspection) or that the organization in some way sponsors civic activism. As we noted in Chapter Two, we sought to include studies that may capture more grassroots mobilization and civic engagement. However, the majority of the current peer-reviewed studies do not yet assess the causal links between this type of engagement and health outcomes.

As we did in Chapter Three, we organize this chapter by types of health outcome, including physical health, behavioral health, healthy behaviors, and mental health. However, we also include the domain of well-being because the nonvoting, civic engagement literature is more robust in illuminating the civic engagement–well-being association than the voting literature. There were a handful of articles that compared civic engagement between different health outcomes. We included the relevant parts of those articles in sections covering the appropriate health outcomes. There has also been focused attention on civic engagement in the adolescent population, which we summarize separately. Finally, as with the voting literature, the overwhelming majority of studies are at the individual level. However, we present articles on community-level outcomes near the end of the chapter.

Civic Engagement and Physical Health

We begin with studies that explore the relationship between physical health and civic engagement.

Self-Rated Health

As we did in Chapter Three, we begin this discussion with 15 studies of self-rated health. Because the outcome indicators in these studies are essentially the same, we organized our findings by region of the world. Overall, these studies suggest a mostly positive relationship between civic engagement and general health, but with some exceptions.

First, we summarize work from the United States. Danso (2017) used cross-sectional data from the 2011–2012 California Health Interview Survey that focused on 42,935 adult immigrants and native-born Americans. Social capital was defined by measures of neighborhood safety, neighborhood trust, social cohesion, and civic engagement, specifically volunteer work. Volunteering was significantly associated with higher levels of immigrant and nonimmigrant health. Similarly, in Pillemer et al. (2010), which is discussed later in this chapter, the authors defined civic engagement as volunteering in an environmental organization or any group concerned with the environment, pollution, and related issues. Using data from the 1974 and 1994 versions of the Alameda County Study (n = 6928), the authors prospectively analyzed the association between 1974 volunteerism and self-rated health outcomes in 1994. They found a positive association between environmental volunteering and self-rated health.

The evidence is largely similar in studies from the Commonwealth countries. For example, Habibov and Weaver (2014) analyzed data from Statistics Canada's General Social Survey, a cross-sectional survey administered in 2008. Civic participation was measured by self-reported voting, and social participation was measured by participation in groups or organizations. All indicators of social capital (including both civic and social participation) were found to be positively and significantly associated with self-rated health. Similarly, Buck-McFadyen et al. (2018) examined cross-sectional data from Canada's 2013 General Social Survey (n = 7,187), finding that self-rated physical health was associated with high trust in institutions, sense of belonging, and civic engagement (defined as volunteering, attending a public meeting, expressing views to a newspaper or politician, and participating in community groups).[1]

Turning to the UK, Emerson et al. (2014) conducted a cross-sectional analysis comparing 279 adults with an intellectual disability with 22,927 adults without an intellectual disability, using data from Understanding Society, a longitudinal survey of adults in the UK. The authors found that higher levels of social and civic participation (defined as organization memberships and social activities with friends) were associated with more positive self-rated health for those both with and without intellectual disabilities.

Similarly, four studies from Europe and Scandinavia lend additional support to the linkage between civic engagement and better self-reported health. Hyyppä and Mäki's (2001) cross section of bilingual adults in Finland (Swedish-speaking and Finnish-speaking) (n = 1284) found that social capital, having friends, and membership in a reli-

---

[1]   The civic engagement index used included voting as one small part.

gious association were positively associated with self-rated health. Similarly, Poortinga's (2006) cross-sectional multilevel analysis of 42,358 observations from 22 countries from the 2002–2003 European Social Survey found that social trust and civic participation (membership participation or volunteering for various organizations) were strongly associated with better self-rated health at the individual level. However, aggregate levels of civic participation at the national level were not associated with individual-level health, leading the author to conclude that "rather than having a contextual influence on health, the beneficial properties of social capital can be found at the individual level." Similarly, a global analysis of adults older than age 50 by Van Groezen, Jadoenandansing, and Pasini (2011), using data from the 2004 Survey on Health, Aging and Retirement and the World Value Survey, found that civic participation (measured by the sum of days per month spent on activities like coursework, volunteering, sports, religious, political or community activities) was positively associated with self-reported health in all countries, and the effect is similar across countries, even when controlling for actual health status and health behaviors. Finally, Grav et al.'s (2013) cross-sectional analysis of data on 235,797 adult survey respondents in the Nord-Trøndelag Health Study 3 (2006–2008) in Norway found that participation in meetings, music, church, outdoor activities, dance, and sports were all related to higher levels of self-rated health.[2]

Findings from Africa, however, are decidedly mixed. Chola and Alaba's (2013) analysis of cross-sectional data from the 2008 South Africa National Income Dynamics Survey (n = 13,381) found positive associations between individual and neighborhood level social capital (including civic participation and social trust and neighborhood social capital) and self-rated health. This finding differed by province; each province varies by administrative system, landscape, climate, economy, population, and language. However, there did not appear to be specific types of provinces in which these relationships were systematically weaker or stronger, leading the authors to recommend adopting interventions that reflect neighborhood-level differences and call for

---

[2]   These outcomes were modeled as a multinomial logistic regression.

more research into specific mechanisms of influence. Avogo (2013) used data from a 2001 survey administered in southern Ghana (n = 1,283) to explore the cross-sectional relationship between social capital (e.g., support from the organization, social control by the organization, participation in organizational activities, and two measures around the organization's encouragement of family planning and HIV/AIDS prevention) and self-rated health. The analysis found that direct civic participation was not associated with better self-rated health. Similarly, Ramlagan, Peltzer and Phaswana-Mafuya (2013) failed to find a significant relationship between civic engagement and self-reported health in an analysis of 3,480 adults older than age 50 from the 2008 Study of Global Aging and Adults Health.

Although most studies provide some evidence of a positive association between self-rated health and various measures of civic engagement, there were some null and contrary findings reported in the literature. For instance, Veenstra's (2000) analysis of 534 observations from a 1997 cross-sectional study of adults in Saskatchewan, Canada, found that an engagement index (including voting, writing letters to editors, and paying attention to community issues) was not associated with self-rated health. Similarly, Petrou and Kupek (2008) conducted a cross-sectional, logistic regression analysis of 13,753 observations from the 2003 Health Survey for England, and found that measures of trust, social support and participation in organizations were all associated with lower self-rated health. Finally, Van Woerden and colleagues' (2011) analysis of 2007 cross-sectional survey data (n = 223) in London found that civic participation, defined as participation in activities of 14 types of organizations, was associated with a lower likelihood of poor self-rated health. The association was unchanged when other social support variables (e.g., marriage, employment, home ownership) were controlled, leading the authors to suggest that other factors can compensate for the benefits of civic participation.

Other Health and Health Care Outcomes

Five studies examine the linkage between civic engagement and various combinations of specific health outcomes, such as disease-related mortality, measured objectively rather than subjectively. For example, a study by Veenstra (2002) found that higher social capital (as measured by aggregating "associational and civic participation by individuals and the density of associational life") was associated with lower mortality. Ziersch et al. (2009), by contrast, took a more general approach to measuring physical health, using the SF-12 (a scale measuring quality of life-related health) in a cross-sectional analysis of 2,013 South Australian survey participants collected in 2003. Their analysis found that higher social capital (e.g., social networks, trust in people, governments and businesses, and reciprocity), cohesion, and civic activities (e.g., picking up trash in public spaces, joining groups, attending protests) was associated with better physical health for urban residents but not for those living in rural areas.

Other studies focused on individual health outcomes. For example, Burr, Han, and Tavares (2016) examined data from the 2004 and 2006 waves of the U.S.-based Health and Retirement Study (n = 7,803) to assess the linkages between cardiovascular disease risk in those participants who were 51 years and older. Using logistic regression in this longitudinal study, the authors found that middle-aged volunteers (51–64 years old) were "less likely to have high central adiposity, lipid dysregulation, elevated blood glucose levels, and MetS [metabolic syndrome] compared with non-volunteers" (Burr, Han, and Tavares, 2016). Volunteers who were age 65 and older were less likely to be hypertensive but more likely to have lipid dysregulation than nonvolunteers. Gold et al. (2002), in turn, used cumulative data from the U.S.-based General Social Survey for 1986–1990 (put out by the Centers for Disease Control and Prevention) to study the relationship between teen birth rates and three separate factors—social cohesion, civic engagement, and community trust—in 1991. Given the study's exploratory intent, teen birth rates are included in this section because we consider them a physical health outcome for purposes of this review. In a cross-sectional path analysis, the authors found that social cohesion, civic engagement, and trust mediated the relationship between poverty and income inequality, on the one hand, and teen birth rate, on the other. Finally, Ransome et al. (2016) used data from the 2004 New York Social Indicators Survey to explore the relationship between late HIV diagnosis and civic engagement, political participation, social cohesion, and informal social control. In a cross-sectional analysis of 2,199 men and women with HIV diagnoses, the highest political participation was associated with lower late HIV diagnosis, independent of income inequality.

Civic Engagement and Behavioral and Mental Health

We turn next to studies of the relationship between civic engagement, health behaviors, and mental and cognitive health.

Health Behaviors

There were four articles in our review that covered health behaviors, including physical activity, alcohol use, and drug use. Although methods vary and civic engagement is defined differently across these health behaviors, civic engagement is associated with positive health behaviors in each instance.

The first two articles explored the linkages between civic engagement and physical activity. Marquez et al. (2016) examined data from a cohort of 335 Latinos who completed the San Diego Prevention Research Center's Household Community Survey in 2009, finding that involvement in various religious, health, neighborhood, professional, social welfare, political, or arts groups was related to having a larger social network. This, in turn, was associated with greater awareness of physical activity resources in the community, which predicted meeting the national physical activity recommendation of 150 minutes per week. Similarly, Pillemer et al. (2010) used longitudinal data from the 1974 and 1994 versions of the Alameda County Study (n = 6,928) to examine the relationship between volunteering in an environmental organization in 1974 and volunteerism and physical activity outcomes in 1994. The authors found that volunteering with environmental organizations and other types of volunteering in midlife significantly predicted the health behavior of self-reported physical activity. Interestingly, environmental volunteering was a stronger predictor for physical activity than "other volunteering," perhaps because environmental volunteering could require more-active outdoor engagement. Two additional articles on health behaviors and civic engagement are described in the section on adolescents later in this chapter.

Mental and Cognitive Health

There are ten studies in this review that look at the association between civic engagement and various indicators of mental health, from self-reported mental health to diagnosed depression and even suicide. Although most studies show a link between better mental health and engagement, some of the findings are mixed.

A few studies focus on depression or depressive symptoms. Pillemer et al. (2010) (discussed in the health behavior section above) also looked at depression as an outcome. Depression was measured using an 18-item scale, and the authors found a positive effect for environmental volunteering and depression. In another study, Taylor (2016) examined cross-sectional data on 184 participants from the Caribbean coast of Colombia and found that depression intensified the association between (1) civic engagement and past political violence exposure and between (2) civic engagement and social trust.

Other studies have failed to find a clear link between depression and civic engagement. A 2013 analysis of cross-sectional data on 3,840 individuals older than age 50 from the first wave of a national survey in South Africa conducted in 2008 found that depressive symptoms (measured by one question about feeling sad, low, or depressed in the past 30 days) were associated with lower social capital (including measures of "social action" and "civic engagement") (Ramlagan, Peltzer, and Phaswana-Mafuya, 2013). However, there was no association between depression symptoms and civic engagement. In another study of a cross section of 13,469 respondents in the South African National Income Dynamics Study, there was no association between participation in any of 18 civic groups or associations and depression, as measured by the ten-item Center for Epidemiologic Studies Depression Scale (Tomita and Burns, 2013). Civic participation was used as an individual-level social capital predictor in this study, and it was defined as participation in any of 18 groups or associations. The findings were null for civic participation.

Moving to more-general mental health outcomes, Bertotti et al. (2013) examined cross-sectional data ($n = 4214$) from a study of 40 neighborhoods in London collected from 2011 to 2012. The authors found that "structural social capital" (including volunteering and attendance at events/activities) was associated with lower rates of Common Mental Disorder (CMD) (a group of mental disorders including anxiety and depression) after controlling for sociodemographic variables. CMD was measured using the General Health Quesionnaire-12, which includes three constructs of anxiety, social dysfunction, and loss of confidence. Similarly, Buck-McFayden et al.'s (2018) analysis of a cross section of 7,187 respondents to Canada's 2013 General Social Survey found trust in people, trust in institutions, civic engagement, and social network size to be associated with good self-reported mental health. Moreover, the aforementioned Australian study by Ziersch et al. (2009) found that civic activities were associated with good self-reported mental health for both urban and rural residents. Finally, a longitudinal analysis by Ding, Berry, and O'Brien (2015) provided an opportunity to better understand the causal links between civic engagement and mental health. In an analysis of 2006–2011 data ($n = 9,498$) from a panel within the Household, Income and Labor Dynamics in Australia Survey, better mental health predicted more community participation in the next year. Greater prior community participation (using a 12-item index that includes informal social connectedness, civic engagement, and political participation) was linked to better mental health the next year independent of initial mental health.

In the area of cognitive health, there are limited studies. However, the aforementioned study by Ramlagan, Peltzer, and Phaswana-Mafuya (2013) found that participants who were 50–69 years old (compared with those over 69 years of age) and who had higher education levels, wealth, and social capital (which in this study included civic engagement) had better cognitive functioning as measured on a battery of cognitive assessments that tested verbal recall, verbal fluency, and digit span.

Other studies have focused on smaller subpopulations. For example, Leedahl, Sellon, and Gallopyn (2017) examined the link between civic participation (group participation, resident council participation, volunteering, and voting in a recent election) and emotional well-being (using the Geriatric Depression Scale) in a sample of 139 older adult nursing home residents in Kansas. The authors also measured social network size, social trust, and social support. Using logistic regression, the authors found that emotional well-being and social support were associated with participation in both groups and resident councils. Similarly, Bergstresser, Brown, and Colesante (2013) conducted a qualitative analysis using focus groups in New York City with 52 people from 2008–2009, about half of whom were black and were self-reported users of mental health services. The goal was to describe user attitudes about political engagement. The focus groups revealed that political participation is connected to social inclusion. The researchers also noticed a theme of political participation "as a component of empowerment for minority groups in general."

Finally, a study by Acevedo, Ellison, and Xu (2014) suggests that the effect of civic engagement on health can be indirect. In a 2004 cross-sectional survey of 1,504 adults in Texas, the authors found that secular civic engagement (involvement in 13 different types of community activities, from voting to tutoring to contacting government) was not directly associated with psychological distress. However, they found that civic engagement significantly buffers the deleterious effects of perceived financial hardship on respondents' levels of psychological distress. Civic engagement does not moderate the effect of residents' perceptions of neighborhood disadvantage (i.e., of factors that create barriers) on psychological distress.

Civic Engagement and Well-Being

Another group of eight studies examined the linkage between civic engagement and well-being, including both general and more-specific conceptualizations of well-being. Although several studies find a clear civic engagement–well-being link, the evidence is somewhat mixed.

Beginning with studies in the United States, Wray-Lake and team explored the relationship between civic engagement and well-being in a cross section of 276 U.S. college students in 2014 and 2015. The team found that both a composite measure of civic engagement (including helping, pro-environmental behavior, volunteering, and charitable giving), and two individual measures of civic engagement (helping and pro-environmental behavior) were each associated with higher well-being (using the 24-item Basic Needs Satisfaction Scale). However, no effects were found for volunteering or charitable giving.

Collins and Guidry (2018) took a slightly different tack, hypothesizing that social capital and civic engagement might mediate the relationship between economic inequality and sense of safety (which we categorize as a form of well-being) in a cross section of 20,271 households in U.S. cities using the 2008 and 2010 Soul of the Community survey. The authors defined civic engagement as activities intended to address community issues, and they operationalized social capital as informal social relationships and interactions. Using structural equation modeling in this cross-sectional analysis, the authors found that those who reported lower civic engagement (including participation in local organizations) also reported feeling less safe, and those in communities with higher inequality reported lower levels of social capital.

Turning to Europe, Cicognani et al. (2015) studied 835 Italian adolescents and young adults, ages 16 to 26, to explore the relationship between involvement in volunteer, youth, religious, and recreational groups and social well-being, as well as the mediating role of sense of community and empowerment. Social well-being was measured using the Mental Health Continuum Short Form. The authors found that group membership, other than in recreational groups, is associated with higher social well-being both directly and when mediated by one's sense of community and empowerment. Similarly, in a 2003 cross-sectional study of 556 Italian adolescents ages 14 to 19, Albanesi, Cicognani and Zani (2007) found that involvement in formal groups is associated with increased civic involvement and an increased sense of community. Furthermore, a sense of community, in turn, predicted social well-being and explains some of the association between civic engagement and social well-being. This suggests that the link between civic engagement and well-being could be mediated by other factors. These empirical linkages are also borne out in work from Goth and Småland (2014), in which interviews with 14 volunteers working on historic vessels in Norway in 2009 suggested that "volunteering in a context of skilled, group-bonded, culturally prestigious activity adds considerably to social capital among elderly men in Norway." However, a study by Serrat et al. (2017) of 182 Spanish adults ages 65 and older failed to find a difference in eudaemonic well-being (measured using the Purpose of Life and Personal Growth subscales of the Ryff Scales of Psychological Well-Being) between a group of 97 active members of political associations and 85 members of a comparison group who were enrolled in university programs but not involved in political organizations.

The cross-sectional nature of the aforementioned studies, however, limits our ability to determine whether the empirical linkages between civic engagement and well-being reflect some underlying causal mechanism. However, there are a few longitudinal studies that allow us to examine questions of causality more closely and explore the role of civic engagement in the life cycle. Fang et al. (2018) explored associations between involvement in organizations and happiness in a longitudinal data set from Canada ($n = 690$), with data collected in 1989, 1992, 1999, and 2010. Using autoregressive cross-lagged models, the authors found consistent associations between higher happiness and higher future civic engagement. The authors found no evidence of a causal pathway from civic engagement to happiness, nor was there evidence for a bidirectional association. The authors concluded that happiness predicts future civic engagement "across the transition to adulthood and into midlife." Finally, Callina et al. (2014) used growth mixture modeling for responses from 1,432 U.S. youths in the 4-H Study of Positive Youth Development. They found that the group in which hopeful future expectations remained moderate across waves and trust decreased significantly and then rose (i.e., were most discrepant from each other across the study) and had the strongest association with high scores on a "contribution" scale that included community leadership, service, helping behaviors, and ideologies. The implications of the findings are somewhat unclear, and the authors call for future research to examine hope-trust trajectories.

Civic Engagement and Adolescents

The topic of adolescent civic engagement has been a focus of a few national and international studies on adolescent behaviors and, therefore, can provide some general findings about the relationship between individual and community characteristics, including individual, family, and social variables and civic participation. Eight studies focused on adolescents in this review.

The Health Behaviour in School-Aged Children Survey (undated) has been used to understand individual and school-level predictors of youth civic engagement. In an analysis of tenth-graders from five countries, Lenzi et al. (2012) found that perceived neighborhood social capital was positively correlated with participation in community organizations. In fact, social environment variables (including family affluence and democratic school climate) were more significant at an aggregate level rather than an individual one. In a study of Italian eighth-graders, Manganelli, Lucidi, and Alivernini (2015) also found that a mix of contextual and individual factors mattered. The authors observed that civic engagement self-efficacy fostered a greater expectation to participate in civic activities. Like other studies linking sense of community with civic engagement, further study among a sample of Italian high school students showed links between sense of community, civic engagement, and social well-being (Albanesi, Cicognani, and Zani, 2007). Sense of community was linked to social well-being and might help explain part of the association between civic engagement and social well-being.

Studies of adolescents in the United States have also explored individual, family, and social variables. One such study (also discussed above) demonstrated that civic engagement and mental health are related. In their analysis of National Longitudinal Survey of Adolescent Health data, Wray-Lake et al. (2017) found that community engagement has mental health benefits for youths, but that depressive symptoms can decrease the likelihood of voting behavior later in life. Another set of analyses from the same study showed that increases in school and family capital was positively associated with later civic engagement (Mahatmya and Lohman, 2012). This finding holds up in other studies using this longitudinal data set. Duke et al. (2009) found that a stronger connection to family and community during adolescence predicted greater likelihood of voting, community volunteer service, involvement in social action groups, and a better sense of civic trust. At a broader contextual level, exposure to community violence depressed the likelihood of community participation among youths (Chen, Propp, and Lee, 2014).

Two other articles looked at alcohol use and civic engagement in adolescents. A 2007 article from Bartkowski and Xu uses cross-sectional data from the 1996 Monitoring the Future study (n = 1,493) of U.S. high school seniors and focuses on the effect of secular civic engagement. The authors conclude that civic engagement in secular organizations—defined as participation in the school newspaper or yearbook, performing arts, organized sports, academic or other clubs, or student government—is associated with less drug use, including alcohol, marijuana, and other illicit drugs. In the second article, Finlay and Flanagan (2013) conducted a latent class analysis of data from the 1970 British Cohort Study (n = 14,025) and found that 16-year-olds who were more involved in sports, volunteering, religious services, and school activities were more likely to be civically engaged in adulthood and were less likely to have problems with alcohol use.

Civic Engagement and Community Health

As with voting studies, the majority of published research is at the individual level—that is, the effects of individual-level civic engagement on individual-level health outcomes. However, we did locate three studies that directly address whether the types of linkages described above scale to the community or regional levels.

For example, Zhu (2017) analyzed pooled, cross-sectional–time-series data on 3,024 continental U.S. counties in the 48 contiguous U.S. states from 1996–2009 to assess the relationship between measures of health equity and various measures of civic activism, including membership of civic clubs, working for a political party or candidate, contributions to public television or radio stations, actively working as a nonpolitical volunteer, and the number of nonprofit organizations per 1,000 population. The analysis found that although increases in racial diversity were related to higher degrees of inequality in access to health care, higher levels of civic engagement (and other forms of structural social capital) were related to lower levels of health care inequality. Therefore, the author concluded that social capital (operationalized through community organizational life, engagement in public affairs, and community volunteerism) can counterbalance some of the effects of race on health care inequality.

Lochner et al. (2003), in turn, analyzed 1995 cross-sectional data on 342 Chicago neighborhoods, finding that higher levels of reported neighborhood membership in civic organizations were associated with lower neighborhood death rates (for ages 45–64) for total mortality and heart disease mortality for whites and blacks; no association was found with cancer mortality.

In another study, Cutlip, Bankston, and Lee (2010) looked specifically at suicide counts in rural U.S. counties between 1999 and 2005 ($n = 1,451$). The authors measured civic engagement using voting in the 2000 election if eligible, number of small manufacturing plants, number of civic and social organizations per 1,000 people, number of churches per 1,000 people, and number of family-owned farms per capita. In this cross-sectional analysis, the authors found that lower suicide rates among whites are associated with civically stronger communities. Because the design was cross-sectional, the authors cautioned that "it cannot be inferred directly that the civically active individuals are less likely to commit suicide."

Summary

Unlike voting, which is a fairly specific behavior defined by clear institutional rules and procedures, civic engagement is a term with many possible definitions. Accordingly, the research literature on broader civic engagement examines a variety of specific civic engagement behaviors. Moreover, this literature is even more international in character, with an even smaller proportion of studies based on data from U.S. contexts. With some exceptions, the general conclusion across nations is that there is an association between positive self-reported health and participation in civic activities. In addition, there is evidence that social capital mediates the relationship between civic engagement and health. In the area of health behaviors specifically, civic engagement is protective against such risk factors as substance use and lack of physical activity. In most cases, good mental health appears to be associated with greater civic participation. Like the voting literature, much of the evidence comes from analysis of cross-sectional data sets. However, there are some longitudinal studies, especially for the adolescent population, that provide the benefit of data sets that allow researchers to track the association between civic engagement and health over time. As with voting, there are a limited number of community-level analyses, but the few studies that do exist suggest the protective benefits of civic engagement in the context of health inequality and health equity. More research is needed that specifically examines the role of community, historical, and structural factors and their roles in influencing nonvoting civic engagement and links to health.

CHAPTER FIVE

Evidence on Civic Engagement-Oriented Interventions

In this chapter, we summarize evidence from a handful of studies that evaluate the effects of interventions designed to promote civic engagement and/or to help realize the health benefits of engaging civically. We include only studies that explicitly seek to estimate an intervention's effects. Therefore, we do not seek to include the full range of studies that describe such interventions or their implementation. Most of the evaluation studies focus on the health effects to individual participants. Also, unlike much of the literature referenced in previous chapters, most of the intervention studies were conducted in the United States. Although the literature on intervention effectiveness is limited, it does point to promising avenues for further program evaluation, particularly how these interventions might work across diverse social and demographic contexts in the United States.

Civic Engagement Interventions to Improve Physical Health

We located several studies evaluating interventions that use civic engagement to improve physical health. Brown et al. (2017) used a quasi-experimental pre-post study design to evaluate civic engagement as an intervention strategy to improve heart health in 23 black women in Boston, Massachusetts. The intervention entailed creating Change Clubs in four churches, where members "met weekly for six months and participated in a step-by-step process using the civic engagement approach" to help build individual and group capacity for engaging civically. The intervention included a three-month planning phase that focused on group unity, determining community need, leadership skills, and developing action plans, followed by a three-month action phase during which the group carried out its action plan. In addition to this civic engagement curriculum, a cardiovascular disease prevention curriculum called Strong Women–Healthy Hearts was also adapted and implemented with this group. Data collection included a pre-post survey of participants to understand demographics, acceptability, and satisfaction with the program. Civic engagement was measured using the Civic Engagement Scale. Health outcomes measured included diet (via two 24-hour dietary recalls), physical activity (via accelerometers) the Rockport One Mile test, blood pressure, height, weight, waist circumference, and body fat percentage. These data were collected two weeks prior to the start of the Change Club and again six months afterward. Researchers also conducted two interviews in each group, one with the leader and one with a member. Study authors found that there was a statistically significant improvement in participants' finish times on the cardiorespiratory fitness test and in their systolic blood pressure. The authors conclude that the study demonstrated "evidence of preliminary effectiveness of using a civic engagement approach to address behavior change in a way that is appealing and acceptable to black women" (Brown et al., 2017).

In another study, Dabelko-Schoeny, Anderson, and Spinks (2010) piloted an intervention in 2008 in a Midwestern city in the United States to promote civic engagement in adults with functional limitations. Subjects came from a convenience sample recruited from two adult day health centers ($N = 43$). The authors compared participants receiving the civic engagement intervention with those receiving treatment as usual. The intervention was a five-session program that included education about the community group they would serve, service (assembling care packages for community groups), and recognition (where participants gave the packages to the community group and received a completion certificate and celebration). The research team collected pre- and post-intervention data regarding purpose, from the Purpose in Life subscale from the Ryff Psychological Well-Being Scale,[1] on a feeling of usefulness, self-esteem, and self-rated health. Participants receiving the intervention reported higher, yet nonsignificant, levels of purpose in life, self-esteem, and perceived physical health compared with those in the control group. However, participants reported a significant decrease in self-esteem and perceived physical health five weeks after the intervention was terminated. The authors caution that this was a pilot study with a small sample size that prevented them from conducting more-sophisticated analyses of the data.

Finally, Wass et al. (2017) examined the effects of existing voter facilitation instruments. The researchers used six rounds of the European Social Survey data—approximately 240,000 individual-level observations from participants in 30 European countries between 2002 and 2013—to examine the relationship among voter turnout, self-reported health conditions (including functional ability), and voter facilitation instruments. The voter facilitation instruments included in the survey were in-person advance voting, holiday or weekend voting, number of election days, postal voting, proxy voting, and voting outside of polling stations. Instead of the expected increase in turnout as a result of increased voter facilitation instruments, the authors found that voter facilitation interacted negatively with self-reported poor health and poor functional ability in countries where the greatest efforts were made to include voters with health-related and functional ability difficulties. Because the analysis was cross-sectional, it is difficult to determine the causality. However, the authors suggested that the relationship might reflect that countries where there is low turnout from people with poor health or poor functional ability are more likely to implement voter facilitation efforts, such as proxy voting, therefore calling into question the causal effects of these participation-increasing measures.

---

[1]   More information on this scale is available online at the Positive Psychology Center's website (undated).

Civic Engagement Interventions to Improve Health Behavior

Two studies evaluated an intervention designed to address behavioral health issues. Wagenaar et al. (2000) conducted a pilot of a program called Communities Mobilizing for Change on Alcohol with the goal of reducing underage youth access to alcohol consumption in a randomized, 15-community trial in the Midwestern United States in 1992 with a follow-up in 1995. The two-and-a-half-year intervention consisted of the following community engagement strategies and efforts: 1,518 one-on-one meetings with community stakeholders and community members to build relationships and understand community dynamics, a review of alcohol policies, development of a strategy team, media advocacy efforts, and policy changes. Data were collected through in-school surveys (n = 3,694 with data at both ninth-grade and 12th-grade time points), telephone surveys of 18–20-year-olds (n = 1,721 with data at both time points) and alcohol retailers (n = 273 off-sale retailers and n = 229 on-sale retailers in 1992), and direct testing of alcohol outlets sales to young customers. Mixed-model regression using the community as the unit of interest found that the intervention had little effect on adolescents but did have a significant effect on behaviors of 18–80-year-olds, who were less likely to provide alcohol to teens and were less likely to buy or drink alcohol. The study was also one of only two we located that explicitly sought to assess the effects of a civic engagement intervention on community policies. The authors found that there was also a significant change in alcohol retailer practices and concluded that "community organizing is a useful intervention approach for mobilizing communities for institutional and policy change to improve the health of the population" (Wagenaar et al., 2000).

Another study that addresses changes in community policy was Subica et al.'s (2016) analysis of a three-year community organizing–based intervention conducted by 21 community organization grantees across the United States between 2009 and 2013. The goal of the intervention was to increase children's healthy food and access to safe recreation opportunities. Researchers conducted interviews quarterly and six months after the intervention to understand "environmental and policy changes resulting from grantee interventions." Authors found that grantees achieved 72 policy wins, a mean of 3.4 per community organization. The policies fell into six policy domains with both direct effects on obesity (such as child nutrition policies) and indirect effects (such as affordable housing). The authors concluded that community organizing–based interventions designed and led by community stakeholders could identify environmental and policy solutions to address structural inequities related to childhood obesity.

Civic Engagement Interventions to Improve Well-Being

Finally, we located several studies that evaluated the effects of civic engagement interventions on well-being more generally across a relatively wide variety of populations. First, a group of researchers in London (Bolton et al., 2016) piloted a community organizing social support group intervention (which included both a support group and a community organizing group) in 2013 with 15 women who were pregnant or had an infant younger than 2 years old. Trained community organizers helped facilitate mothers' support groups and provided six workshops about community organizing, parenting, and child health. The authors measured effectiveness using the 12-item General Health Questionnaire, the 14-item Warwick-Edinburgh Mental Well-Being Scale, and an adapted Social Capital questionnaire in a pre-post evaluation design. Authors found no change in well-being, but they found increases in social capital and reductions in distress for women in the support group.

The remainder of the studies focused on interventions in the United States. For example, MacPhee et al. (2017) conducted an evaluation study of the Family Leadership Training Institute (FLTI) in Colorado to understand its effects on civic knowledge, empowerment, civic engagement, and community health. The intervention entailed personal leadership skill development and then ten weeks of civic engagement modules, followed by a community-based civic capstone project to address a community, health, or education issue. Using a sample of 847 FLTI participants and 166 comparison adults, researchers conducted pre- and post-design surveys. Measures included civic literacy and empowerment, along with civic knowledge using questions about state laws, budgets, and civic engagement, which was measured by activities and voting. They also measured social network and community connectedness, which are important for individual well-being. The authors found short-term effects in civic literacy, empowerment, and civic engagement. Eighty-six percent of FLTI graduates sustained meaningful levels of civic engagement, which included leadership, advocacy, program implementation and involvement in media campaigns, and after-program completion. The authors concluded that this type of family empowerment model can foster both civic engagement and relationships with diverse constituents.

Turning to youth populations, Beaudoin, Thorson, and Hong (2006) conducted an evaluation of a public health media campaign that aimed to promote social support among youths. The authors argue that youths with more social support and meaningful participation are more healthy in general. Conducted in Kansas, the campaign started in 1998, targeted adults, and provided information about and encouraged positive youth interactions, advocated improved perceptions of the role of youths in communities, and included newspaper and TV outlets. The campaign ran for two years and was adjusted after year one. The research team measured civic perceptions (e.g., social trust, friends concerned about youths in Kansas) and civic participation (e.g., membership in eight types of organizations) as components of social capital (n = 614 in 1998); researchers found that civic perceptions increased over the course of the campaign yet civic engagement did not change.

Varma et al. (2015) focused on Experience Corps, which promotes civic engagement among older adults through school-based volunteer activities, such as group tutoring or helping out at the school library. The authors explored the experience of 46 members of Experience Corps in Baltimore, Maryland, using focus groups in 2015. Focus group administrators asked about stressors and rewards associated with the volunteer experience, which could be regarded as a general measure of well-being. Stressors included managing behavior problems, such as physical aggression in children, but interpersonal and personal rewards from volunteering, such as facilitating improvement in a child, balanced those stressors.

Finally, Bloemraad and Terriquez (2016) examined how community-based organizations (CBOs) can inspire and maintain a culture of engagement and health in marginalized populations. Using survey and interview data from the Building Healthy Communities Initiative in 2013–2015 ($N = 1,210$ participants in youth civic groups at 68 CBOs in low-income, immigrant communities in California), the researchers examined CBO ability to develop individual civic capacity and efficacy, build social networks, and create a shared commitment to collective well-being. The authors found that CBOs can both generate individual well-being effects and reduce structural barriers to good health by supporting civic capacity and a sense of efficacy.

Summary

We located ten studies that provide empirical evaluations of interventions that use civic engagement principles and practices to improve physical health, health behavior, and well-being (see Table 5.1). There appears to be limited evidence of effects on physical health and mixed evidence of effects on health behavior and well-being. As with the studies reviewed earlier in the report, most of the evidence relates to impacts on individuals. However, one study found effects on community policy and practice. As we summarize in Table 5.1, the target populations vary in demographic background; therefore, more work is needed to determine how well these interventions might work across a more-diverse population mix.

Table 5.1
Summary of Findings from Intervention Studies

Intervention	Target Population	Outcomes Addressed	Evidence
Change Clubs (Brown et al, 2017)	Black women	Diet, physical activity, and various biometric measures	Improvement in cardiorespiratory fitness, blood pressure
Community service (Dabelko-Schoeny, Anderson, and Spinks, 2010)	Adults with functional limitations	Feelings of usefulness, self-esteem, and self-rated health	Nonsignificant improvements at post-test; decline in self-esteem and self-rated health at a five-week follow-up
Voter facilitation instruments (Wass et al., 2017)	European adults	Self-reported health conditions and voter turnout	Voter facilitation efforts appear to be adopted by countries with high concentrations of those with poor functioning, but no clear evidence of causal effects.
Communities Mobilizing for Change on Alcohol (Wagenaar et al., 2000)	Youths	Alcohol consumption and behaviors and underage retail sales	No effect on adolescents; significant reductions in young adults' provision of alcohol to minors
Community organizing (Subica et al., 2016)	Obese children	Environmental and policy changes	Grantees achieved 72 policy changes, with direct and indirect effects on obesity
Community organizing and social support (Bolton et al., 2016)	Pregnant and postpartum women	General health, mental well-being, and social capital	Improvements in social capital, reductions in distress, no change in well-being

Table 5.1—Continued

Intervention	Target Population	Outcomes Addressed	Evidence
Family Leadership Training Institute (MacPhee et al., 2017)	Adult FLTI participants	Civic literacy, civic knowledge, civic engagement, and voting	Short-term improvements in civic literacy, empowerment, and engagement; sustained effects of civic engagement
Public health media campaign (Beaudoin, Thorson, and Hong, 2006)	Youths	Civic perceptions, civic participation, and social capital	Civic perceptions increased; civic engagement did not change
Experience Corps, Baltimore, Maryland (Varma et al., 2015)	Older adults	Stressors and rewards from volunteering	Stressors were balanced by interpersonal and personal rewards from the experience
Role of CBOs in civic capacity (Bloemraad and Terriquez, 2016)	Youths	Individual well-being	CBOs can generate individual well-being effects in youth civic groups

CHAPTER SIX

Discussion

Civic engagement is identified in the Culture of Health Action Framework as one of the key drivers for Action Area 1 (Making Health a Shared Value). The driver can serve as a mechanism for translating changes in a health-related mindset and sense of community into tangible actions that could lead to new partnerships, improvements in the health conditions found in communities, and the degree of integration among health services and systems. However, the evidence base linking civic engagement and health has not previously been examined in a systematic way. The purpose of this report was to summarize the current evidence, with a particular focus on drawing out any literature showing causal links between civic engagement and health. As noted earlier and at the end of this chapter, there are limitations in the current empirical base in terms of both cultural context in which studies are conducted and how civic engagement is defined and operationalized, which can also vary by social and historical context. In this chapter, we return to the questions posed at the beginning of the report, summarize key findings, and identify some primary gaps in knowledge.

Is There an Empirical Relationship Between Health and Civic Engagement?

The majority of studies meeting our selection criteria found that increases in physical and mental health and well-being are related to increases in civic engagement, whether through voting or through such activities as volunteering and membership in civic organizations. These findings held across various health outcomes, including self-reported health, physical disability, various aspects of mental health, the prevalence of healthy behaviors, and (in some cases) specific health conditions (see Table 6.1). Similarly, the health–civic engagement linkage applied to various forms of civic engagement, including voting, membership in community organizations, volunteering, secular activism through churches, and others. Our findings were also consistent regardless of study design quality, including longitudinal, cross-sectional (with statistical controls), and qualitative studies (see Table 6.1).

A few studies suggest that the effects of poor health on civic engagement are cumulative, both with multiple conditions (Sund et al., 2016) and with illnesses that last many years (Mattila et al., 2018). However, the nature and the strength of the linkage varied, in some cases, among specific conditions—e.g., those with cancer sometimes were shown to be more prone to civic action than those with other medical conditions. Our findings also come from various regions of the world, including North America, Europe, Australia, and Africa.

This finding of a link between civic engagement and health, although quite consistent across studies, is not universal, as some null findings are reported in the published literature (e.g., Van Groezen, Jadoenandansing, and Pasini, 2011; Veenstra, 2000; Ramlagan, Peltzer, and Phaswana-Mafuya, 2013) and other studies report inconsistent

Table 6.1
Number of Studies for Each Health Outcome and Type of Civic Engagement

Health Outcome	Voting	Civic Engagement
Physical health	10	20
Mental health	9	13
Patient populations		2
Community health	4	4
Well-being	0	9
Adolescents	0	8

findings (e.g., Chola and Alaba, 2013) (see Table 6.2). Moreover, as with any scientific summary of evidence, it is unclear whether publication bias has led to the underreporting of other null findings. Nevertheless, the basic conclusion supported by this review is that the research to date links better health with more civic engagement.

As noted in Chapter Two, we elected to include non-U.S. sources in our review, believing it best to assess the consistency of findings across national contexts by comparing the findings. As noted in Table 6.2, the overall findings are a bit more supportive of the health–

Table 6.2
Number of Studies by Key Finding (U.S. vs. Non-U.S. Sources)

	Location		Method			All Studies
	U.S.	Non-U.S.	Qualitative	Cross-Sectional	Longitudinal[a]	
Civic engagement linked to better health	19	29	4	34	10	48
No connection found	0	3	0	2	1	3
Civic engagement moderates linkage of other variables with health	3	1	0	4	0	4
Mixed findings	2	0	0	0	2	2
Youths	2	3	0	3	2	5
Health related to candidate preference	2	0	0	1	1	2
Total	28	36	4	44	16	64

[a] Counts include one retrospective pre-post study, in which a cross section of respondents were asked to recount changes over time.

civic engagement linkage in studies from non-U.S. contexts than U.S. contexts (81 percent versus 68 percent). This difference, although not large given the small number of studies overall, could be due to differences in culture, population demographics, and (as noted below) differences in institutional characteristics. On the whole, however, the picture painted by U.S. literature and non-U.S. literature is similar.

Is Health a Cause of Civic Engagement, a Consequence of It, or Both?

Most of the studies we located relied on cross-sectional data sets, thus, limiting our ability to assess whether empirical relationships are truly causal, discern whether good health increases civic engagement, or vice versa. However, there are a few longitudinal studies suggesting that poor health earlier in life is associated with lower levels of civic engagement later in life (Ojeda and Pacheco, 2017; Wray-Lake et al., 2017). Moreover, the effects of poor health seem to work in both directions— i.e., early depression is associated with less engagement later in life; and early civic engagement is associated with less depression later in life. There is evidence that the effects can persist over long periods of time (Pillemer et al., 2010). This has led some authors to speculate that health and civic engagement make up a reinforcing feedback loop. As Ojeda (2015) notes:

> (1) individuals with depression are unlikely to participate in the political process, (2) the lack of participation leads to underrepresentation and a lack of policies that benefit those with depression, and (3) the lack of beneficial policy outcomes perpetuates the experience of depression. And so it repeats.

If true, and depending on the strength of any such effect, those with good health initially might accrue additional influence in the political process over time, although those with poor health initially might become increasingly disconnected from politics. This dynamic could contribute to increasing inequities over time. However, we emphasize that empirical evidence for such a cycle is preliminary.

What Causal Mechanisms Link Civic Engagement and Health?

The studies reviewed provide little direct evidence about what types of causal mechanisms might support observed associations between civic engagement and health. Nonetheless, many provide informed speculation based on theory and prior literature. We can obtain additional insight by relating the findings to some classic theories of political participation from the political science, political sociology, and political psychology literature, which have been built up over decades of research.

Typical explanations of variation in voter participation rates can be grouped into several categories. The simplest, although most controversial, is the *rational actor* theory, which holds that individuals are dispassionate utility-maximizers who vote if the perceived benefits exceed perceived costs. Generally, the benefits of participating include the perceived value of the good at stake (e.g., individual or community health), the perceived likelihood that policy changes or other collective action can help, and the private benefits (e.g., satisfaction) of participating (Lubell, Zahran, and Vedlitz, 2007). The private costs of participating include such factors as time off from work, transportation, hiring babysitters, and others. The problem is that the benefits are discounted by the extremely small probability that a single individual's participation will change the collective decision, which means that the private costs will dominate the rational actor decision and the individual will decide not to participate. From this perspective, even the comparatively low voter participation rates in the United States are surprising, leading researchers in this tradition to talk about the "paradox of voting"(Downs, 1957). The *resource model* (Verba and Nie, 1972), although not wholly inconsistent with the rational model, holds that variations in socioeconomic status—which is a proxy for variations in free time, education, and knowledge of the voting systems— allows some people to bear the costs of voting more successfully and to more likely understand the broader potential benefits.

Some of the evidence summarized here is generally consistent with this viewpoint—for example, physical disability, which may increase the private costs and burdens of participation, has been shown in some studies to be related to lower voting turnout (Schur et al., 2002), which (barring robust mail-in voting options) requires physical presence at the polls. However, we did not locate any studies that examined the resource burdens of private costs associated with caring for others, which seems likely to affect the individual decision calculus about whether and how much to engage civically. Alternatively, it might be that such considerations are genuinely less important than other factors.

For other schools of thought, however, voting is a more-nuanced phenomenon. The *psychological model*, for instance, focuses on variations in a range of individual-level factors, such as attitudes and dispositions (e.g., altruism, shyness, efficacy, and conflict avoidance), skills (e.g., language proficiency) (Bobo and Gilliam, 1990; Leighley and Vedlitz, 1999), and other factors such as gender (Inglehart and Norris, 2003), race, and ethnicity that are often correlated with such attitudes. Traditionally, party identification has been viewed as an individual-level cognitive and emotive "filter" through which individuals perceive the benefits and costs of voting (Huckfeldt and Sprague, 1992), though there is ample evidence that party loyalty is decreasing across many democracies.

As noted above, one study (Albright et al., 2015) speculates that lower rates of civic engagement among smokers might result from, among other things, a sense of grievance given the increasing social stigma against smoking. Moreover, it seems likely that depression may might affect how individuals make decisions about participation in civic life.

By contrast, there is more existing evidence related to what is often termed as the *sociological model*. This perspective emphasizes social context, including the influence of spouses and other household members (Hobbs, Christakis, and Fowler, 2014; Wolfinger and Wolfinger, 2008), social networks (Gerber, Green, and Larimer, 2008; McClurg, 2003), and interpersonal trust, all of which are shaped by broader processes of political socialization through childhood and into adulthood (Jennings and Niemi, 2014).

Indeed, some studies explain the linkage between health and civic engagement by the fact that poor health can lead to increased social isolation, often because of difficulties in getting around or in social stigma. Although most explicit discussions of this mechanism were studies of physical health, it is reasonable to suspect that the same also holds for mental health; one study (Ojeda and Pacheco, 2017) describes how mental health problems might interrupt the normal process of political socialization during the late teen and early adult years. There is reason to believe that stigma can apply to health behaviors, such as smoking (Albright et al., 2015; Denny and Doyle, 2007). However, the nature of this relationship might be mediated by culture, as is suggested by the finding that heavy smokers (but not heavy drinkers) have lower rates of civic engagement in Ireland because of its pub culture (Denny and Doyle, 2007).

Finally, the *institutional model* focuses on the "rules of the game" embedded in electoral systems, including voting registration rules, the use of concurrent local-national elections, the drawing of voting districts, and other factors (Highton, 2017). For the most part, the studies summarized earlier do not address variations in institutional configurations. Nonetheless, the fact that a study of the United States finds lower rates of engagement among those with physical disabilities (Schur et al., 2002) while a study from Scandinavia (Söderland and Rapeli, 2015) does not find the same lower rates might reflect differences in voting procedures and other features of political institutions. At least one study, moreover, suggests that, when considering institutional designs, we should weigh not just mechanisms for articulating political preferences but also the broader aspects of the political economy, such as industry concentration, which might influence opportunities to affect the practices of private organizations with influence over the health-related conditions of communities (Cutlip, Bankston, and Lee, 2010; Mactaggart et al., 2017).

Finally, a handful of studies explore the role of civic engagement as a factor that moderates the relationship between health and other variables. One study suggests that civic engagement mediates the link between income inequality and teen birth rates (Gold et al., 2002), while another finds that secular civic engagement might buffer the effects of financial difficulty on psychological distress (Acevedo, Ellison, and Xu, 2014).

Is the Nature of the Health–Civic Engagement Relationship Different Across Various Segments of the Population?

The relatively small number of studies for each health–civic engagement measure limits our confidence in the precision of the magnitude of effects for any one category, and differences in specific measures limit the ability to draw comparisons across conditions. Nonetheless, several studies made explicit comparisons among health conditions. For example, there is evidence that those with cancer are more likely to vote than those with heart disease, a difference the authors attribute to social stigma around heart disease and to stronger political organization around cancer (Gollust and Rahn, 2015). Another study found that being a member of an organization is associated with lower death rates from heart disease but not from cancer (Lochner et al., 2003). There is also some evidence that the nature of the health–civic engagement connection might vary by social group, as blacks with low education and cancer are more likely to turn out than well-educated whites with cancer (Gollust and Rahn, 2015).

Important Gaps in the Literature

Aside from voting, which is clearly defined, there appears to be a lack of clear agreement in terminology and constructs for measuring civic engagement. This definitional discordance was clear in the literature reviewed for this report. Some studies treat civic engagement as an aspect of social capital, while other studies focus on specific activities, such as participating in formal organizations, volunteering with community organizations or at community events, donating blood, and others. A small number of studies address participation in religious organizations. Other studies focus less on activities and more on mindsets, such as attitudes toward political participation. Moreover, the literature is quite global in nature, with a healthy number from the United States, but a little more than half from Europe, Africa, and Commonwealth countries.

Although studies of the linkages between civic engagement and physical health are most common, followed by mental health, there is a relative dearth of studies seeking to link civic activism to broader concepts of well-being (see Table 6.1). Perhaps more important is the fact that the vast majority of studies focus on the individual level, both in the measurement of civic engagement and in health outcomes. Indeed, the articles we located examine links between civic engagement and self-reported health, mental health (both general and specific conditions), suicide, drug and alcohol use, risk factors for cardiac disease, physical activity, and general well-being. Several compare the civic engagement-health connection across health conditions. However, there is much less attention to whether individual-level engagement is related to community health and to the community level conditions (e.g., infrastructure, policies) that shape health.

Finally, we located a handful of evaluations of civic engagement–related interventions designed to address health outcomes, each providing evidence of positive effects. Interestingly, two such studies addressed the effects of the interventions on policy changes in the community. However, for most studies, the focus was on health effects for participating individuals only.

CHAPTER SEVEN

Next Steps for the Robert Wood Johnson Foundation and the Field

Our review of literature on the linkages between civic engagement (both voting and other forms) and health found evidence of connections between the two and preliminary indications that health is both a cause and a consequence of civic engagement. More research is needed that leverages longitudinal designs to unpack causal relationships and further elucidate how health experience and voting behavior evolve over time. In addition, further analyses on how the health status of a community, and not simply an individual, relates to voting participation would provide useful information on the role of the relationship among enfranchisement, participation, health equity, and positive health outcomes.

Given the analysis above, the following are next steps that the RWJF and other funders might consider:

- **Improve the availability and analysis of robust longitudinal and multilevel data sets.** Research in this area requires merging data sets on health with those on voting and other forms of civic engagement, which would create an extra hurdle for researchers. Funders should consider supporting the creation, maintenance, and analysis of thorough, longitudinal data sets to further understand the mechanisms underlying the health–civic engagement link. Among these linkages is the relationship between individual- and community-level phenomena—e.g., between individual-level engagement and community-level health, between community-level depression and individual-level engagement, and others. Given the impracticality of randomization, such longitudinal and/ or multilevel analysis are likely to provide the best practical ways to better understand the causal dynamics involved. Moreover, as part of such an effort, funders might support efforts to promote harmonization in terminology and data definitions related to various forms of civic engagement (not related to voting).

- **Support more research that specifically targets causal mechanisms.** Several studies provide evidence that one of the key mechanisms linking health and civic engagement might be social connectivity—that is, in the role of poor health disrupting social networks that support engagement in community and public life. Conversely, civic engagement might itself promote or nurture social ties that help support good health. More research to understand this and other causal mechanisms would be useful in designing interventions.
- **Support research that examines how civic engagement influences structural and systemic barriers to health.** As noted at the outset of this report, our study was not focused on how civic engagement can influence upstream drivers of health or changes in the social and economic environment to promote better health outcomes. This does not mean that this is not an area that could benefit from more investigation. There is a broader body of work on civic engagement and collective action, but the challenge is how to link that work to proximal and distal determinants of health. Furthermore, exploration of the pathways by which civic engagement changes equity-based policies, environments, and community power structures (and, in turn, can be *causally* linked to health outcomes) is needed.
- **Support the development and sustainment of multidisciplinary communities of practice.** Similarly, work in this area involves an ability to blend expertise and perspectives from public health and from political science, sociology, and other social/behavior sciences. This, in turn, might impede the development of shared concepts, frameworks, and other factors needed to nurture a strong community of scholarly practice. We expect

that there is more study of civic engagement underway, but not all of this research is reaching the peer-reviewed literature. Funders should consider sponsoring conferences, forums, and networks to provide venues in which researchers can collaborate (including around shared data sets, as mentioned above) and more actively contribute articles to build the literature base on health–civic engagement relationship.

- **Support collaborative intervention design within communities of practice.** As noted above, the number of evaluations of interventions remains limited. Sound intervention design requires knowledge of potential causal mechanisms that might be leveraged; practical knowledge of how to design and implement cost-effective, feasible interventions; and the evaluation capacity needed to systematically track implementation and assess causality. Support for forums involving individuals and organizations with these various skill sets might help speed up the process of identifying ways to both promote civic engagement and realize any related health benefits.

- **Support the investigation into how health-related civic engagement relates to efforts to improve community health.** The summary above examined civic engagement in general. However, it is possible that civic engagement specifically focused on health issues could be more likely to lead to collective action to improve community health. Furthermore, the current literature does not yet have enough specificity on how different forms of civic engagement operate, outside of voting. That is, more work is needed to understand mechanisms underlying community organizing, advocacy, social mobilization, and other forms of participation and the relative effect on health outcomes.

Data Abstraction Form

Author:

Year Published:

Journal:

Categorization: *(i.e., voting or other)*

Country/Region:

Subpopulation: (*e.g. women, youth)*

Year Data Collected:

Civic Engagement Measured:
(e.g., voting, organizing)

Health Outcomes Measured:
(include definitions)

Sample Size, Description:

Method to Assess Causal Relationships:

Key Findings:

Proposed Causal Mechanisms/Theory:

Notes:

Articles Reviewed

Author (Year)	Title
Abbott (2010)	"Social Capital and Health: The Role of Participation"
Abu-Ras (2013)	"American Muslim Physicians' Public Role Post-9/11 and Minority Community" "Empowerment: Serving the Underserved"
Acevedo, Ellison, and Xu (2014)	"Is It Really Religion? Comparing the Main and Stress-Buffering Effects of Religious and Secular Civic Engagement on Psychological Distress"
Albanesi, Cicognani, and Zani (2007)	"Sense of Community, Civic Engagement and Social Well-Being in Italian Adolescents"
Albright et al. (2016)	"Smoking and (Not) Voting: The Negative Relationship Between a Health-Risk Behavior and Political Participation in Colorado"
Amnå (2012)	"How Is Civic Engagement Developed Over Time? Emerging Answers from a Multidisciplinary Field"
Avogo (2013)	"Social Capital, Civic Engagement, and Self-Rated Health in Ghana"
Balsano (2005)	"Youth Civic Engagement in the United States: Understanding and Addressing the Impact of Social Impediments on Positive Youth and Community Development"
Bartkowski and Xu (2007)	"Religiosity and Teen Drug Use Reconsidered. A Social Capital Perspective"
Bazargan, Kang, and Bazargan (1991)	"A Multivariate Comparison of Elderly African Americans and Caucasians Voting Behavior: How Do Social, Health, Psychological, And Political Variables Effect Their Voting?"
Beaudoin, Thorson, and Hong (2006)	"Promoting Youth Health by Social Empowerment: A Media Campaign Targeting Social Capital"

Author (Year)	Title
Bergstresser, Brown, and Colesante (2013)	"Political Engagement as an Element of Social Recovery: A Qualitative Study"
Bertotti et al. (2013)	"Types of Social Capital and Mental Disorder in Deprived Urban Areas: A Multilevel Study of 40 Disadvantaged London Neighbourhoods"
Bhatti and Hansen (2012)	"Retiring from Voting: Turnout Among Senior Voters"
Blakely, Kennedy and Kawachi (2001)	"Socioeconomic Inequality in Voting Participation and Self-Rated Health"
Block et al. (2012)	"Food Sovereignty, Urban Food Access, and Food Activism: Contemplating the Connections Through Examples from Chicago"
Bloemraad and Terriquez (2016)	"Cultures of Engagement: The Organizational Foundations of Advancing Health in Immigrant and Low-Income Communities of Color"
Bolton et al. (2016)	"Community Organizing and Community Health: Piloting an Innovative Approach to Community Engagement Applied to an Early Intervention Project in South London"
Booth (2016)	"Civic Engagement Builds Capacity for Health Departments"
Borges (2010)	"Social Capital and Self-Rated Health Among Adolescents in Brazil: An Exploratory Study"
Bosquet (2009)	"The Vote of Acute Medical Inpatients: A Prospective Study"
Brettle (1995)	"Do Nursing Home Residents Use the Right to Vote?"
Brown (2017)	"Improving Heart Health Among Black/African American Women Using Civic Engagement: A Pilot Study"
Brown et al. (2003)	"The Health Politics of Asthma: Environmental Justice and Collective Illness Experience in the United States"
Buck-McFadyen (2018)	"Social Capital and Self-Rated Health: A Cross-Sectional Study of the General Social Survey Data Comparing Rural and Urban Adults in Ontario"
Bulanda and Jendrek (2016)	"Grandparenting Roles and Volunteer Activity"
Burr, Han, and Tavares (2016)	"Volunteering and Cardiovascular Disease Risk: Does Helping Others Get 'Under the Skin?'"

Author (Year)	Title
Bynner, Schuller, and Feinstein (2003)	"Wider Benefits of Education: Skills, Higher Education and Civic Engagement"
Callina et al. (2014)	"Hope in Context: Developmental Profiles of Trust, Hopeful Future Expectations, and Civic Engagement Across Adolescence"
Cené et al. (2011)	"Understanding Social Capital and HIV Risk in Rural African American Communities"
Chan and Chiu (2007)	"The Politics of Citizenship Formation: Political Participation of Mental Health Service Users in Hong Kong"
Chandra et al. (2016)	"Drivers of Health as a Shared Value: Mindset, Expectations, Sense of Community, and Civic Engagement"
Chen, Propp, and Lee (2014)	"Connection Between Adolescent's Exposure to Community Violence and Future Civic Engagement Behaviors During Their Young Adulthood"
Choi et al. (2014)	"Social Capital, Mortality, Cardiovascular Events and Cancer: A Systematic Review of Prospective Studies"
Chola and Alaba (2013)	"Association of Neighbourhood and Individual Social Capital, Neighbourhood Economic Deprivation and Self-Rated Health in South Africa—A Multi-Level Analysis"
Cicognani et al. (2015)	"Sense of Community and Empowerment Among Young People: Understanding Pathways from Civic Participation to Social Well-Being"
Collins and Guidry (2018)	"What Effect Does Inequality Have on Residents' Sense of Safety? Exploring the Mediating Processes of Social Capital and Civic Engagement"
Corburn (2014)	"Civic Innovation, Deliberation, and Health Impact Assessment: Democratic Planning and Civic Engagement in San Francisco"
Cutler, Hendricks, and O'Neill (2011)	"Civic Engagement and Aging"
Cutlip, Bankston, and Lee (2010)	"Civic Community and Nonmetropolitan White Suicide"
Dabelko-Schoeny, Anderson, and Spinks (2010)	"Civic Engagement for Older Adults with Functional Limitations: Piloting an Intervention for Adult Day Health Participants"
Danso (2017)	"Immigrant Health Disparities: Does Neighborliness Improve Health?"

Author (Year)	Title
Denny and Doyle (2007)	"Analysing the Relationship Between Voter Turnout and Health in Ireland"
Denny and Doyle (2007)	". . . Take Up Thy Bed, and Vote: Measuring the Relationship Between Voting Behaviour and Indicators of Health"
Ding, Berry, and O'Brien (2015)	"One-Year Reciprocal Relationship Between Community Participation and Mental Wellbeing in Australia: A Panel Analysis"
Duke et al. (2009)	"From Adolescent Connections to Social Capital: Predictors of Civic Engagement in Young Adulthood"
Emerson et al. (2014)	"Perceptions of Neighbourhood Quality, Social and Civic Participation and the Self-Rated Health of British Adults with Intellectual Disability: Cross-Sectional Study"
Fang et al. (2018)	"Happiness Is the Way: Paths to Civic Engagement Between Young Adulthood and Midlife"
Finlay and Flanagan (2013)	"Adolescents' Civic Engagement and Alcohol Use: Longitudinal Evidence for Patterns of Engagement and Use in the Adult Lives of a British Cohort"
Fowler and Dawes (2008)	"Two Genes Predict Voter Turnout"
Fowler, Baker, and Dawes (2008)	"Genetic Variation in Political Participation"
Gele and Harsløf (2012)	"Barriers and Facilitators to Civic Engagement Among Elderly African Immigrants in Oslo"
Gold et al. (2002)	"Teen Births, Income Inequality, and Social Capital: Developing an Understanding of the Causal Pathway"
Gollust and Rahn (2015)	"The Bodies Politic: Chronic Health Conditions and Voter Turnout in the 2008 Election"
Goth and Småland (2014)	"The Role of Civic Engagement for Men's Health and Well-Being in Norway: A Contribution to Public Health"
Gottlieb and Gillespie (2008)	"Volunteerism, Health, and Civic Engagement Among Older Adults"
Grav et al. (2013)	"Association of Personality, Neighbourhood, and Civic Participation with the Level of Perceived Social Support: The HUNT study, a Cross-Sectional Survey"
Gray, Khoo, and Reimondos (2012)	"Participation in Different Types of Volunteering at Young, Middle and Older Adulthood"

Author (Year)	Title
Habibov and Weaver (2014)	"Endogenous Social Capital and Self-Rated Health: Results from Canada's General Social Survey"
Hart, Matsuba, and Atkins (2014)	"Civic Engagement and Child and Adolescent Well-Being"
Hylton (2018)	"The Role of Civic Literacy and Social Empathy on Rates of Civic Engagement Among University Students"
Hyyppä and Mäki (2001)	"Individual-Level Relationships Between Social Capital and Self-Rated Health in a Bilingual Community"
Johnson and Lee (2017)	"Factors Associated with Volunteering Among Racial/Ethnic Groups: Findings from the California Health Interview Survey"
Kannan and Veazie (2018)	"Political Orientation, Political Environment, and Health Behaviors in the United States"
Kaskie et al. (2008)	"Civic Engagement as a Retirement Role for Aging Americans"
Kelleher et al. (2002)	"Indicators of Deprivation, Voting Patterns, and Health Status at Area Level in the Republic of Ireland"
Kelly (2014)	"Voting and Mental Illness: The Silent Constituency"
Kelly and Nash (2018)	"Voter Participation Among People Attending Mental Health Services in Ireland"
Kuehl, Drury, and Anderson (2015)	"Civic Engagement and Public Health Issues: Community Support for Breastfeeding Through Rhetoric and Health Communication Collaborations"
Lancee and ter Hoeven (2010)	"Self-Rated Health and Sickness-Related Absence: The Modifying Role of Civic Participation"
Leedahl, Sellon, and Gallopyn (2017)	"Factors Predicting Civic Engagement among Older Adult Nursing Home Residents"
Lenzi et al. (2012)	"Family Affluence, School and Neighborhood Contexts and Adolescents' Civic Engagement: A Cross-National Study"
Lerner et al. (2002)	"Positive Youth Development: Thriving as the Basis of Personhood and Civil Society"
Levitt (2008)	"Religion as a Path to Civic Engagement"
Lewis, MacGregor, and Putnam (2013)	"Religion, Networks, and Neighborliness: The Impact of Religious Social Networks on Civic Engagement"
Liggett et al. (2014)	"Results of a Voter Registration Project at 2 Family Medicine Residency Clinics in the Bronx, New York"

Author (Year)	Title
Lochner et al. (2003)	"Social Capital and Neighborhood Mortality Rates in Chicago"
Longhi and Canton (2011)	"Reflections on Citizenship and Barriers to Popular Participation in the Unified Health System"
López-Cevallos et al. (2013)	"Strengthening Rural Latinos' Civic Engagement for health: The Voceros de Salud Project"
Lopez and Marcelo (2008)	"The Civic Engagement of Immigrant Youth: New Evidence from the 2006 Civic and Political Health of the Nation Survey"
Lyson, Torres, and Welsh (2001)	"Scale of Agricultural Production, Civic Engagement, and Community Welfare"
MacPhee et al. (2017)	"Promotion of Civic Engagement with the Family Leadership Training Institute"
Mactaggart et al. (2017)	"Exploring the Determinants of Health and Wellbeing in Communities Living in Proximity to Coal Seam Gas Developments in Regional Queensland"
Mahatmya and Lohman (2012)	"Predictors and Pathways to Civic Involvement in Emerging Adulthood: Neighborhood, Family, and School Influences"
Mahmood, Vaughn, and Tyuse (2014)	"Gender Disparity in Civic Engagement Among Former Offenders in the U.S. Population"
Maloney, Van Deth, and Roßteutscher (2008)	"Civic Orientations: Does Associational Type Matter?"
Manganelli, Lucidi, and Alivernini (2014)	"Adolescents' Expected Civic Participation: The Role of Civic Knowledge and Efficacy Beliefs"
Manganelli, Lucidi, and Alivernini (2015)	"Italian Adolescents' Civic Engagement and Open Classroom Climate: The Mediating Role of Self-Efficacy"
Marlowe, Bartley, and Hibtit (2014)	"The New Zealand Refugee Resettlement Strategy: Implications for Identity, Acculturation and Civic Participation"
Marquez et al. (2016)	"Latino Civic Group Participation, Social Networks, and Physical Activity"
Martinez et al. (2011)	"Invisible Civic Engagement Among Older Adults: Valuing the Contributions of Informal Volunteering"

Author (Year)	Title
Martinson and Minkler (2006)	"Civic Engagement and Older Adults: A Critical Perspective"
Marum (1988)	"Rural Community Organizing and Development Strategies in Alaska Native Villages"
Mattila et al. (2013)	"Healthy Voting: The Effect of Self-Reported Health on Turnout in 30 Countries"
Mattila et al. (2018)	"Sick Leave from Work and the Voting Booth? A Register-Based Study on Health and Turnout"
McAllister (2008)	"Public Support for Democracy: Results from the Comparative Study of Electoral Systems Project"
McBride (2006)	"Civic Engagement, Older Adults, and Inclusion"
Minkler (2012)	"Community Organizing and Community Building for Health and Welfare: Third Edition"
Minkler and Wallerstein (2012)	"Improving Health Through Community Organization and Community Building: Perspectives from Health Education and Social Work"
Mino et al. (2011)	"Associations Between Political/Civic Participation and HIV Drug Injection Risk"
Montague and Eiroa-Orosa (2018)	"In It Together: Exploring How Belonging to a Youth Activist Group Enhances Well-Being"
Morrow-Howell and Freedman (2006)	"Introduction: Bringing Civic Engagement into Sharper Focus"
Morrow-Howell, O'Neill, and Greenfield (2011)	"Civic Engagement: Policies and Programs to Support a Resilient Aging Society"
Myroniuk, Prell, and Kohler (2017)	"Why Rely on Friends Instead of Family? The Role of Exchanges and Civic Engagement in a Rural Sub-Saharan African Context"
Nissen (2010)	"Political Activism as Part of a Broader Civic Engagement: The Case of SEIU Florida Healthcare Union"
Obach and Tobin (2014)	"Civic Agriculture and Community Engagement"
Ojeda (2015)	"Depression and Political Participation"

Author (Year)	Title
Ojeda and Pacheco (2017)	"Health and Voting in Young Adulthood"
Okamoto (2017)	"'It's Like Moving the Titanic:' Community Organizing to Address Food (In)Security"
Ott, Heindel, and Papandonatos (2003)	"A Survey of Voter Participation by Cognitively Impaired Elderly Patients"
Pastor, Terriquez, and Lin (2018)	"How Community Organizing Promotes Health Equity, and How Health Equity Affects Organizing"
Petrou and Kupek (2008)	"Social Capital and Its Relationship with Measures of Health Status: Evidence from the Health Survey for England 2003"
Pillemer et al. (2010)	"Environmental Volunteering and Health Outcomes over a 20-Year Period"
Poortinga (2006)	"Social Capital: An Individual or Collective Resource for Health?"
Prainsack (2011)	"Voting with Their Mice: Personal Genome Testing and the 'Participatory Turn' in Disease Research"
Prewitt et al. (2014)	"Civic Engagement and Social Cohesion: Measuring Dimensions of Social Capital to Inform Policy"
Ramlagan, Peltzer, and Phaswana-Mafuya (2013)	"Social Capital and Health Among Older Adults in South Africa"
Ransome et al. (2016)	"Social Capital Is Associated with Late HIV Diagnosis: An Ecological Analysis"
Reitan (2003)	"Too Sick to Vote? Public Health and Voter Turnout in Russia During the 1990s"
Renick et al. (2005)	"A Civic Engagement Paradigm for Reforming Health Administration Education and Recreating the Community"
Serrat (2017)	"Older People's Participation in Political Organizations: The Role of Generativity and Its Impact on Well-Being"
Seyfang (2003)	"Growing Cohesive Communities One Favour at a time: Social Exclusion, Active Citizenship and Time Banks"
Shin and McCarthy (2013)	"The Association Between County Political Inclination and Obesity: Results from the 2012 Presidential Election in the United States"

Author (Year)	Title
Söderlund and Rapeli (2015)	"In Sickness and in Health"
Stefaniak, Bilewicz, and Lewicka (2017)	"The Merits of Teaching Local History: Increased Place Attachment Enhances Civic Engagement and Social Trust"
Subica et al. (2016)	"Community Organizing for Healthier Communities: Environmental and Policy Outcomes of a National Initiative"
Sund et al. (2016)	"How Voter Turnout Varies Between Different Chronic Conditions? A Population-Based Register Study"
Tang, Choi, and Morrow-Howell (2010)	"Organizational Support and Volunteering Benefits for Older Adults"
Taylor (2016)	"Impact of Political Violence, Social Trust, and Depression on Civic Participation in Colombia"
Tolbert et al. (2002)	"Civic Community in Small-Town America: How Civic Welfare Is Influenced by Local Capitalism and Civic Engagement"
Tolbert, Lyson, and Irwin (1998)	"Local Capitalism, Civic Engagement, and Socioeconomic Well-Being"
Tomita and Burns (2013)	"A Multilevel Analysis of Association Between Neighborhood Social Capital and Depression: Evidence from the First South African National Income Dynamics Study"
Torney-Purta (2013)	"A Psychological View of Civic Engagement Augmented by Introducing the Developmental Niche Model: Essay Review of Teenage Citizens: The Political Theories of the Young by Constance A. Flanagan"
Touchton, Sugiyama, and Wampler (2017)	"Democracy at Work: Moving Beyond Elections to Improve Well-Being"
Tyler (2007)	"Developing Prosocial Communities Across Cultures"
Uppal and Larochelle-Côté (2012)	"Factors Associated with Voting"
Urbatsch (2017)	"Influenza and Voter Turnout"
Väänänen et al. (2009)	"Engagement in Cultural Activities and Cause-Specific Mortality: Prospective Cohort Study"
van Groezen, Jadoenandansing, and Pasini (2011)	"Social Capital and Health Across European Countries"

Author (Year)	Title
Van Woerden et al. (2011)	"The Relationship of Different Sources of Social Support and Civic Participation with Self-Rated Health"
Varma et al. (2015)	"Experience Corps Baltimore: Exploring the Stressors and Rewards of High-Intensity Civic Engagement"
Veenstra (2000)	"Social Capital, SES and Health: An Individual-Level Analysis"
Veenstra (2002)	"Social Capital and Health (Plus Wealth, Income Inequality and Regional Health Governance)"
Veenstra and Lomas (1999)	"Home Is Where the Governing Is: Social Capital and Regional Health Governance"
Viswanath, Steele, and Finnegan, Jr. (2006)	"Social Capital and Health: Civic Engagement, Community Size, and Recall of Health Massages"
Wagenaar et al. (2000)	"Communities Mobilizing for Change on Alcohol: Outcomes from a Randomized Community Trial"
Wakefield et al. (2001)	"Environmental Risk and (Re)action: Air Quality, Health, and Civic Involvement in an Urban Industrial Neighbourhood"
Wass et al. (2017)	"Voting While Ailing? The Effect of Voter Facilitation Instruments on Health-Related Differences in Turnout"
Weng and Lee (2016)	"Why Do Immigrants and Refugees Give Back to Their Communities and What Can We Learn from Their Civic Engagement?"
Wray-Lake et al. (2017)	"Examining Links from Civic Engagement to Daily Well-Being from a Self-Determination Theory Perspective"
Wray-Lake et al. (2017)	"Examining Associations Between Civic Engagement and Depressive Symptoms from Adolescence to Young Adulthood in a National U.S. Sample"
Wynne (2006)	"Civic Engagement Through Civic Agriculture: Using Food to Link Classroom and Community"
Zhu (2017)	"'Healing Alone?' Social Capital, Racial Diversity and Health Care Inequality in the American States"
Ziegenfuss, Davern, and Blewett (2008)	"Access to Health Care and Voting Behavior in the United States"
Ziersch et al. (2009)	"Social Capital and Health in Rural and Urban Communities in South Australia"

Detailed Findings on Articles Described in Report

The table in this appendix provides additional information on key findings from the 64 research articles selected for inclusion in this report.

Table C.1
Key Findings From Research Articles Used In Report

Author (Year)	Title	Location	Quality Categorization	Health and Well-Being Indicators	Civic Engagement Indicators	Association
Acevedo, Ellison, and Xu (2014)	"Is It Really Religion? Comparing the Main and Stress-Buffering Effects of Religious and Secular Civic Engagement on Psychological Distress"	U.S. (Texas)	Cross-sectional	Psychological distress	Civic engagement	Civic engagement moderates relationship between financial hardship and psychological distress
Albanesi, Cicognani, and Zani (2007)	"Sense of Community, Civic Engagement and Social Well-Being in Italian Adolescents"	Italy	Cross-sectional	Social well-being	Civic engagement	Higher civic engagement related to higher well-being
Albright et al. (2016)	"Smoking and (Not) Voting: The Negative Relationship Between a Health-Risk Behavior and Political Participation in Colorado"	U.S. (Colorado)	Cross-sectional	Smoking	Voting	Nonsmokers more likely to vote than smokers

Table C.1—Continued

Author (Year)	Title	Location	Quality Categorization	Health and Well-Being Indicators	Civic Engagement Indicators	Association
Avogo (2013)	"Social Capital, Civic Engagement, and Self-Rated Health in Ghana"	Africa (southern Ghana)	Cross-sectional	Self-rated health	Civic engagement	Civic engagement not related to better health
Bartkowski and Xu (2007)	"Religiosity and Teen Drug Use Reconsidered: A Social Capital Perspective"	U.S.	Cross-sectional	Alcohol use	Civic engagement	Higher civic engagement related to less alcohol use
Bergstresser, Brown, and Colesante (2013)	"Political Engagement as an Element of Social Recovery: A Qualitative Study"	U.S. (New York City)	Qualitative	Self-reported mental health service users	Civic engagement	Political participation related to social inclusion

Table C.1—Continued

Author (Year)	Title	Location	Quality Categorization	Health and Well-Being Indicators	Civic Engagement Indicators	Association
Bertotti et al. (2013)	"Types of Social Capital and Mental Disorder in Deprived Urban Areas: A Multilevel Study of 40 Disadvantaged London Neighbourhoods"	UK (London)	Cross-sectional	CMD	Civic engagement	Higher civic engagement related to lower rates of CMD
Bhatti and Hansen (2012)	"Retiring from Voting: Turnout Among Senior Voters"	Denmark	Cross-sectional	Hospital days	Voting	Higher civic engagement associated with better health
Blakely, Kennedy, and Kawachi (2001)	"Socioeconomic Inequality in Voting Participation and Self-Rated Health"	U.S. and Finland	Cross-sectional	Influenza	Voting	Influenza outbreaks associated with lower voter turnout
Bosquet (2009)	"The Vote of Acute Medical Inpatients: A Prospective Study"	France (Paris suburbs)	Qualitative	Internal medicine inpatients	Voting	Medical conditions are among the factors cited by inpatients for not voting

Table C.1—Continued

Author (Year)	Title	Location	Quality Categorization	Health and Well-Being Indicators	Civic Engagement Indicators	Association
Buck-McFadyen et al. (2018)	"Social Capital and Self-Rated Health: A Cross-Sectional Study of the General Social Survey Data Comparing Rural and Urban Adults in Ontario"	Canada	Cross-sectional	Self-rated health, self-reported mental health	Civic engagement	Higher civic engagement related to better health
Burr, Han, and Tavares (2016)	"Volunteering and Cardiovascular Disease Risk: Does Helping Others Get 'Under the Skin?'"	U.S.	Longitudinal	Cardiovascular disease risk	Civic engagement	Volunteering associated with better health across some conditions
Callina et al. (2014)	"Hope in Context: Developmental Profiles of Trust, Hopeful Future Expectations, and Civic Engagement Across Adolescence"	U.S.	Longitudinal	Hopeful future expectations, trust	Civic engagement	Mixed

Table C.1—Continued

Author (Year)	Title	Location	Quality Categorization	Health and Well-Being Indicators	Civic Engagement Indicators	Association
Chen, Propp, and Lee (2014)	"Connection Between Adolescent's Exposure to Community Violence and Future Civic Engagement Behaviors During Their Young Adulthood"	U.S.	Longitudinal	Exposure to community violence	Civic engagement	Exposure to violence associated with lower levels of community participation by youths
Chola and Alaba (2013)	"Association of Neighbourhood and Individual Social Capital, Neighbourhood Economic Deprivation and Self-Rated Health in South Africa—A Multi-Level Analysis"	South Africa	Cross-sectional	Self-rated health	Civic engagement	Higher civic engagement related to better health

Table C.1—Continued

Author (Year)	Title	Location	Quality Categorization	Health and Well-Being Indicators	Civic Engagement Indicators	Association
Cicognani et al. (2015)	"Sense of Community and Empowerment Among Young People: Understanding Pathways from Civic Participation to Social Well-Being"	Italy	Cross-sectional	Social well-being	Civic engagement	Higher civic engagement related to higher well-being
Collins and Guidry (2018)	"What Effect Does Inequality Have on Residents' Sense of Safety? Exploring the Mediating Processes of Social Capital and Civic Engagement"	U.S. (urban areas)	Cross-sectional	Sense of safety	Civic engagement	Civic engagement may mediate link between economic inequality and sense of safety
Cutlip, Bankston, and Lee (2010)	"Civic Community and Nonmetropolitan White Suicide"	U.S. (rural counties)	Cross-sectional	Suicide counts	Civic engagement	Higher civic engagement related to lower suicide counts

Table C.1—Continued

Author (Year)	Title	Location	Quality Categorization	Health and Well-Being Indicators	Civic Engagement Indicators	Association
Danso (2017)	"Immigrant Health Disparities: Does Neighborliness Improve Health?"	U.S. (California)	Cross-sectional	Self-rated health	Civic engagement	Civic engagement related to better health
Denny and Doyle (2007)	"Analysing the Relationship Between Voter Turnout and Health in Ireland"	Great Britain	Longitudinal	Self-rated health, smoking, drinking, mental health	Voting	Better health associated with higher voter turnout
Duke et al. (2009)	"From Adolescent Connections to Social Capital: Predictors of Civic Engagement in Young Adulthood"	U.S.	Longitudinal	Connection to family and community	Civic engagement	Stronger family and community connection associated with more civic engagement subsequently

Table C.1—Continued

Author (Year)	Title	Location	Quality Categorization	Health and Well-Being Indicators	Civic Engagement Indicators	Association
Emerson et al. (2014)	"Perceptions of Neighbourhood Quality, Social and Civic Participation and the Self-Rated Health of British Adults with Intellectual Disability: Cross-Sectional Study"	UK	Cross-sectional	Self-rated health	Civic engagement	Higher civic engagement related to better health among those with and without intellectual disabilities
Fang et al. (2018)	"Happiness Is the Way: Paths to Civic Engagement Between Young Adulthood and Midlife"	Canada	Longitudinal	Happiness	Civic engagement	No association between civic engagement and reported happiness

Table C.1—Continued

Author (Year)	Title	Location	Quality Categorization	Health and Well-Being Indicators	Civic Engagement Indicators	Association
Finlay and Flanagan (2013)	"Adolescents' Civic Engagement and Alcohol Use: Longitudinal Evidence for Patterns of Engagement and Use in the Adult Lives of a British Cohort"	Great Britain	Cross-sectional	Alcohol use	Civic engagement	Teen civic engagement associated with civic engagement as adults
Gold et al. (2002)	"Teen Births, Income Inequality, and Social Capital: Developing an Understanding of the Causal Pathway"	U.S.	Cross-sectional	Teen birth rates	Civic engagement	Civic engagement mediates relationship between poverty and teen birth rate
Gollust and Rahn (2015)	"The Bodies Politic: Chronic Health Conditions and Voter Turnout in the 2008 Election"	U.S.	Cross-sectional	Cancer and heart diseases diagnoses	Voting	Cancer patients more likely to vote; heart patients less likely to vote

Table C.1—Continued

Author (Year)	Title	Location	Quality Categorization	Health and Well-Being Indicators	Civic Engagement Indicators	Association
Goth and Småland (2014)	"The Role of Civic Engagement for Men's Health and Well-Being in Norway—A Contribution to Public Health"	Norway	Qualitative	Social capital	Civic engagement	Volunteering in a context of skilled, group-bonded, culturally prestigious activity adds considerably to social capital
Grav et al. (2013)	"Association of Personality, Neighbourhood, and Civic Participation with the Level of Perceived Social Support: The HUNT Study, a Cross-Sectional Survey"	Norway	Cross-sectional	Self-rated health	Civic engagement	Civic engagement related to better health

Table C.1—Continued

Author (Year)	Title	Location	Quality Categorization	Health and Well-Being Indicators	Civic Engagement Indicators	Association
Habibov and Weaver (2014)	"Endogenous Social Capital and Self-Rated Health: Results from Canada's General Social Survey"	Canada	Cross-sectional	Self-rated health	Voting, civic engagement	Civic engagement associated with better health
Hyyppä and Mäki (2001)	"Individual-Level Relationships Between Social Capital and Self-Rated Health in a Bilingual Community"	Finland	Cross-sectional	Self-rated health	Civic engagement	Civic engagement related to better health
Kelleher et al. (2002)	"Indicators of Deprivation, Voting Patterns, and Health Status at Area Level in the Republic of Ireland"	Ireland	Cross-sectional	Self-rated health	Voting	Higher voting rates related to better health

Table C.1—Continued

Author (Year)	Title	Location	Quality Categorization	Health and Well-Being Indicators	Civic Engagement Indicators	Association
Kelly (2014)	"Voting and Mental Illness: The Silent Constituency"	Ireland, Germany, Israel, and Canada	Cross-sectional	Psychiatric inpatients	Voting	Psychiatric inpatients less likely to vote than others
Kelly and Nash (2018)	"Voter Participation Among People Attending Mental Health Services in Ireland"	Ireland	Qualitative	Mental health service consumers	Voting	Explores specific pathways through which health impedes electoral participation
Leedahl, Sellon, and Gallopyn (2017)	"Factors Predicting Civic Engagement Among Older Adult Nursing Home Residents"	Kansas (nursing homes)	Cross-sectional	Emotional well-being	Civic engagement	Civic engagement related to higher well-being
Lenzi et al. (2012)	"Family Affluence, School and Neighborhood Contexts and Adolescents' Civic Engagement: A Cross-National Study"	Belgium, Canada, Italy, Romania, and England	Cross-sectional	Neighborhood social capital	Civic engagement	Civic engagement related to higher rates of social capital

Table C.1—Continued

Author (Year)	Title	Location	Quality Categorization	Health and Well-Being Indicators	Civic Engagement Indicators	Association
Lochner et al. (2003)	"Social Capital and Neighborhood Mortality Rates in Chicago"	U.S. (Chicago)	Cross-sectional	Mortality	Civic engagement	Higher civic engagement related to lower mortality
Mahatmya and Lohman (2012)	"Predictors and Pathways to Civic Involvement in Emerging Adulthood: Neighborhood, Family, and School Influences"	U.S.	Longitudinal	School and family capital	Civic engagement	Increases in school and family capital was positively associated with later civic engagement
Manganelli, Lucidi, and Alivernini (2015)	"Adolescents' Expected Civic Participation: The Role of Civic Knowledge and Efficacy Beliefs"	Italy	Cross-sectional	Self-efficacy	Civic engagement	Civic engagement in school associated with greater expectation to engage civically later in life
Marquez et al. (2016)	"Latino Civic Group Participation, Social Networks, and Physical Activity"	U.S. (San Diego, California)	Cross-sectional	Physical activity	Civic engagement	Higher civic engagement related to more physical activity

Table C.1—Continued

Author (Year)	Title	Location	Quality Categorization	Health and Well-Being Indicators	Civic Engagement Indicators	Association
Mattila et al. (2013)	"Healthy Voting: The Effect of Self-Reported Health on Turnout in 30 Countries"	30 European countries	Longitudinal	Self-reported health	Voting	Better health associated with higher voter turnout
Mattila et al. (2018)	"Sick Leave from Work and the Voting Booth? A Register-Based Study on Health and Turnout"	Finland	Cross-sectional	Multiple illnesses over several years	Voting	Multiple illnesses over time associated with lower voting rates
Mino et al. (2011)	"Associations Between Political/ Civic Participation and HIV Drug Injection Risk"	U.S. (New York City)	Cross-sectional	Substance use and related behaviors (i.e., needle sharing)	Voting	Civic engagement related to higher prevalence of healthy behaviors (e.g., avoiding needle-sharing)
Ojeda (2015)	"Depression and Political Participation"	U.S.	Longitudinal	Depression	Voting	Depression associated with lower rates of participation

Table C.1—Continued

Author (Year)	Title	Location	Quality Categorization	Health and Well-Being Indicators	Civic Engagement Indicators	Association
Ojeda and Pacheco (2017)	"Health and Voting in Young Adulthood"	U.S.	Longitudinal	Self-rated health; depression; physical limitations	Voting	Better self-rated health and mental health associated with higher turnout
Ott, Heindel, and Papandonatos (2003)	"A Survey of Voter Participation by Cognitively Impaired Elderly Patients"	U.S.	Cross-sectional	Dementia	Voting	Higher levels of dementia related to less knowledge about and participation in elections
Petrou and Kupek (2008)	"Social Capital and Its Relationship with Measures of Health Status: Evidence from the Health Survey for England 2003"	UK (England)	Cross-sectional	Self-rated health	Civic engagement	Civic engagement related to lower self-rated health

Table C.1—Continued

Author (Year)	Title	Location	Quality Categorization	Health and Well-Being Indicators	Civic Engagement Indicators	Association
Pillemer et al. (2010)	"Environmental Volunteering and Health Outcomes Over a 20-Year Period"	U.S. (Alameda County, California)	Longitudinal	Self-rated health, physical activity, depression	Civic engagement	Environmental volunteering associated with better health
Poortinga (2006)	"Social Capital: An Individual or Collective Resource for Health?"	Europe (22 countries)	Cross-sectional	Self-rated health	Civic engagement	Civic engagement related to better individual health, but not at the collective level
Ramlagan, Peltzer, and Phaswana-Mafuya (2013)	"Social Capital and Health Among Older Adults in South Africa"	South Africa	Cross-sectional	Self-rated health, depression, cognitive functioning	Civic engagement	Higher civic engagement related to less depression
Ransome et al. (2016)	"Social Capital Is Associated with Late HIV Diagnosis: An Ecological Analysis"	U.S. (New York)	Cross-sectional	HIV diagnosis	Civic engagement	Civic engagement related to lower rates of late HIV diagnosis

Table C.1—Continued

Author (Year)	Title	Location	Quality Categorization	Health and Well-Being Indicators	Civic Engagement Indicators	Association
Schur et al. (2002)	"Enabling Democracy: Disability and Voter Turnout"	U.S.	Cross-sectional	Disabilities	Voting	Physical disability related to lower voter participation
Shin and McCarthy (2013)	"The Association Between County Political Inclination and Obesity: Results from the 2012 Presidential Election in the United States"	U.S.	Cross-sectional	County-level obesity	Voting	Higher obesity related to higher support for Republican presidential candidate
Söderlund and Rapeli (2015)	"In Sickness and in Health"	Denmark, Finland, Iceland, Norway, and Sweden	Cross-sectional	Self-reported health	Voting	Better health associated with higher rates of voting

Table C.1—Continued

Author (Year)	Title	Location	Quality Categorization	Health and Well-Being Indicators	Civic Engagement Indicators	Association
Sund et al. (2016)	"How Voter Turnout Varies Between Different Chronic Conditions? A Population-Based Register Study"	Finland	Cross-sectional	Alcoholism, mental health disorders, chronic diseases	Voting	Increases in number of health conditions associated with decreases in voter participation
Taylor (2016)	"Impact of Political Violence, Social Trust, and Depression on Civic Participation in Colombia"	Colombia (Caribbean coast)	Cross-sectional	Depression	Civic engagement	Depression mediates link between exposure to violence and civic engagement
Urbatsch (2017)	"Influenza and Voter Turnout"	Finland and U.S.	Cross-sectional	Influenza	Voting	Influenza outbreaks associated with lower voter turnout
Van Groezen, Jadoenandansing, and Pasini (2011)	"Social Capital and Health Across European Countries"	10 European and Scandinavian countries	Cross-sectional	Self-rated health	Civic engagement	Civic engagement related to better health

Table C.1—Continued

Author (Year)	Title	Location	Quality Categorization	Health and Well-Being Indicators	Civic Engagement Indicators	Association
Van Woerden et al. (2011)	"The Relationship of Different Sources of Social Support and Civic Participation with Self-Rated Health"	UK (London)	Cross-sectional	Self-rated health	Civic engagement	Civic engagement related to better health
Veenstra (2000)	"Social Capital, SES and Health: An Individual-Level Analysis"	Canada (Saskatchewan)	Cross-sectional	Self-rated health	Civic engagement	Civic engagement not associated with health
Veenstra (2002)	"Social Capital and Health (Plus Wealth, Income Inequality and Regional Health Governance)"	Canada (Saskatchewan)	Cross-sectional	Mortality	Civic engagement	Higher civic engagement related to lower mortality

Table C.1—Continued

Author (Year)	Title	Location	Quality Categorization	Health and Well-Being Indicators	Civic Engagement Indicators	Association
Wray-Lake et al. (2017)	"Examining Associations Between Civic Engagement and Depressive Symptoms from Adolescence to Young Adulthood in a National U.S. Sample"	U.S.	Longitudinal	Depression	Voting	Adolescent and early young adulthood depressive symptoms predict decreases in later voting
Zhu (2017)	"'Healing Alone?' Social Capital, Racial Diversity and Health Care Inequality in the American States"	U.S. (48 contiguous states)	Cross-sectional	Health equity	Civic engagement	Higher civic engagement related to more health equity
Ziegenfuss, Davern, and Blewett (2008)	"Access to Health Care and Voting Behavior in the United States"	U.S.	Retrospective, pre-post	Health care access	Voting	Problems accessing care associated with preference for Democratic candidate

Table C.1—Continued

Author (Year)	Title	Location	Quality Categorization	Health and Well-Being Indicators	Civic Engagement Indicators	Association
Ziersch et al. (2009)	"Social Capital and Health in Rural and Urban Communities in South Australia"	Australia (southern regions)	Cross-sectional	Quality of life-related health, self-reported mental health	Civic engagement	Higher civic engagement related to better health in urban, but not rural, areas

References

Acevedo, G. A., C. G. Ellison, and X. Xu, "Is It Really Religion? Comparing the Main and Stress-Buffering Effects of Religious and Secular Civic Engagement on Psychological Distress," *Society and Mental Health*, Vol. 4, No. 2, 2014, pp. 111–128. As of August 1, 2019:
https://www.scopus.com/inward/record.uri?eid=2-s2.0-84993683714&doi=10.1177%2f2156869313520558&partnerID=40&md5=dd7f811a20f2cf1bd6c98 85c37969418

Albanesi, C., E. Cicognani, and B. Zani, "Sense of Community, Civic Engagement and Social Well-Being in Italian Adolescents," *Journal of Community and Applied Social Psychology*, Vol. 17, No. 5, 2007, pp. 387–406. As of August 1, 2019:
https://www.scopus.com/inward/record.uri?eid=2-s2.0-34948845110&doi=10.1002%2fcasp.903&partnerID=40&md5=ec560851a626eef9bb5e1dafe9eb2a2e

Albright, Karen, Nancy Hood, Ming Ma, and Arnold H. Levinson, "Smoking and (Not) Voting: The Negative Relationship Between a Health-Risk Behavior and Political Participation in Colorado," *Nicotine and Tobacco Research*, Vol. 18, No. 3, 2015, pp. 371–376.

Avogo, W. A., "Social Capital, Civic Engagement, and Self-Rated Health in Ghana," *Etude de la Population Africaine*, Vol. 27, No. 2, 2013, pp. 188–202. As of August 1, 2019:
https://www.scopus.com/inward/record.uri?eid=2-s2.0-84905057688&doi=10.11564%2f27-2-440&partnerID=40&md5=705030165f69f 647449fd1acbabf5274

Ballard, P. J., L. T. Hoyt, and M. C. Pachucki, "Impacts of Adolescent and Young Adult Civic Engagement on Health and Socioeconomic Status in Adulthood," *Child Development*, Vol. 90, No. 4, July 2019, pp. 1138–1154. As of August 1, 2019:
http://www.ncbi.nlm.nih.gov/pubmed/29359473

Bartkowski, J. P., and X. Xu, "Religiosity and Teen Drug Use Reconsidered: A Social Capital Perspective," *American Journal of Preventive Medicine*, Vol. 32, No. 6, Supplement, 2007, pp. S182–S194. As of August 1, 2019: https://www.sciencedirect.com/science/article/pii/S0749379707001420?via%3Dihub

Bazargan, Mohsen, Tai S. Kang, and Shahrzad Bazargan, "A Multivariate Comparison of Elderly African Americans and Caucasians Voting Behavior: How Do Social, Health, Psychological, and Political Variables Effect Their Voting?" *International Journal of Aging and Human Development*, Vol. 32, No. 3, 1991, pp. 181–198.

Beaudoin, C. E., E. Thorson, and T. Hong, "Promoting Youth Health by Social Empowerment: A Media Campaign Targeting Social Capital," *Health Communication*, Vol. 19, No. 2, 2006, pp. 175–182. As of August 1, 2019: https://www.scopus.com/inward/record.uri?eid=2-s2.0-33645960416&doi=10.1207%2fs15327027hc1902_9&partnerID=40&md5=5c2da2d910e7e2c474c9c618fbe2b8e2

Bergstresser, S. M., I. S. Brown, and A. Colesante, "Political Engagement as an Element of Social Recovery: A Qualitative Study," *Psychiatric Services*, Vol. 64, No. 8, 2013, pp. 819–821. As of August 1, 2019: https://www.ncbi.nlm.nih.gov/pmc/articles/PMC4545250/pdf/nihms-700192.pdf

Bertotti, M., P. Watts, G. Netuveli, G. Yu, E. Schmidt, P. Tobi, S. Lais, and A. Renton, "Types of Social Capital and Mental Disorder in Deprived Urban Areas: A Multilevel Study of 40 Disadvantaged London Neighbourhoods," *PLoS ONE*, Vol. 8, No. 12, 2013. As of August 1, 2019: https://journals.plos.org/plosone/article/file?id=10.1371/journal.pone.0080127&type=printable

Bhatti, Yosef, and Kasper M. Hansen, "Retiring from Voting: Turnout Among Senior Voters," *Journal of Elections, Public Opinion and Parties*, Vol. 22, No. 4, 2012, pp. 479–500.

Blakely, Tony A., Bruce P. Kennedy, and Ichiro Kawachi, "Socioeconomic Inequality in Voting Participation and Self-Rated Health," *American Journal of Public Health*, Vol. 91, No. 1, 2001, pp. 99–104.

Bloemraad, I., and V. Terriquez, "Cultures of Engagement: The Organizational Foundations of Advancing Health in Immigrant and Low-Income Communities of Color," *Social Science and Medicine*, Vol. 165, 2016, pp. 214–222.

Bobo, Lawrence, and Franklin D. Gilliam, "Race, Sociopolitical Participation, and Black Empowerment," *American Political Science Review*, Vol. 84, No. 2, 1990, pp. 377–393.

Bolton, M., I. Moore, A. Ferreira, C. Day, and D. Bolton, "Community Organizing and Community Health: Piloting an Innovative Approach to Community Engagement Applied to an Early Intervention Project in South London," *Journal of Public Health (United Kingdom)*, Vol. 38, No. 1, 2016, pp. 115–121.

Bosquet, A., A. Medjkane, D. Voitel-Warneke, P. Vinceneux, and I. Mah, "The Vote of Acute Medical Inpatients: A Prospective Study," *Journal of Aging and Health*, Vol. 21, No. 5, 2009, pp. 699–712. As of August 1, 2019: https://www.scopus.com/inward/record.uri?eid=2-s2.0-67849101066&doi=10.117 7%2f0898264309338297&partnerID=40&md5=812c65d30c2324d3a78ed46e86 17a96f

Brown, A. G. M., L. B. Hudson, K. Chui, N. Metayer, N. Lebron-Torres, R. A. Seguin, and S. C. Folta, "Improving Heart Health Among Black/African American Women Using Civic Engagement: A Pilot Study," *BMC Public Health*, Vol. 17, No. 1, 2017.

Brown, Theodore M., and Elizabeth Fee, "Social Movements in Health," *Annual Review of Public Health*, Vol. 35, 2014, pp. 385–398.

Buck-McFadyen, E., N. Akhtar-Danesh, S. Isaacs, B. Leipert, P. Strachan, and R. Valaitis, "Social Capital and Self-Rated Health: A Cross-Sectional Study of the General Social Survey Data Comparing Rural and Urban Adults in Ontario," *Health and Social Care in the Community*, Vol. 27, 2018. As of August 1, 2019: https://onlinelibrary.wiley.com/doi/pdf/10.1111/hsc.12662

Burr, J. A., S. H. Han, and J. L. Tavares, "Volunteering and Cardiovascular Disease Risk: Does Helping Others Get 'Under the Skin?'" *Gerontologist*, Vol. 56, No. 5, 2016, pp. 937–947. As of August 1, 2019: https://academic.oup.com/gerontologist/article/56/5/937/2605275

Callina, K. S., S. K. Johnson, M. H. Buckingham, and R. M. Lerner, "Hope in Context: Developmental Profiles of Trust, Hopeful Future Expectations, and Civic Engagement Across Adolescence," *Journal of Youth and Adolescence*, Vol. 43, No. 6, 2014, pp. 869–883.

Chandra, Anita, Carolyn E. Miller, Joie D. Acosta, Sarah Weilant, Matthew Trujillo, and Alonzo Plough, "Drivers of Health as a Shared Value: Mindset, Expectations, Sense of Community, and Civic Engagement," *Health Affairs*, Vol. 35, No. 11, 2016, pp. 1959–1963.

Chen, W. Y., J. Propp, and Y. Lee, "Connection Between Adolescent's Exposure to Community Violence and Future Civic Engagement Behaviors During Their Young Adulthood," *Child and Adolescent Social Work Journal*, Vol. 32, No. 1, 2014, pp. 45–55.

Chola, L., and O. Alaba, "Association of Neighbourhood and Individual Social Capital, Neighbourhood Economic Deprivation and Self-Rated Health in South Africa—A Multi-Level Analysis," *PLoS ONE*, Vol. 8, No. 7, 2013.

Cicognani, E., D. Mazzoni, C. Albanesi, and B. Zani, "Sense of Community and Empowerment Among Young People: Understanding Pathways from Civic Participation to Social Well-Being," *Voluntas*, Vol. 26, No. 1, 2015, pp. 24–44.

Collins, C. R., and S. Guidry, "What Effect Does Inequality Have on Residents' Sense of Safety? Exploring the Mediating Processes of Social Capital and Civic Engagement," *Journal of Urban Affairs*, Vol. 40, No. 7, 2018, pp. 1009–1026.

Cornish, Flora, Cristian Montenegro, Kirsten van Reisen, Flavia Zaka, and James Sevitt, "Trust The Process: Community Health Psychology After Occupy," *Journal of Health Psychology*, Vol. 19, No. 1, January 2014, pp. 60–71.

Cutlip, A. C., W. B. Bankston, and M. R. Lee, "Civic Community and Nonmetropolitan White Suicide," *Archives of Suicide Research*, Vol. 14, No. 3, 2010, pp. 261–265.

Dabelko-Schoeny, H., K. A. Anderson, and K. Spinks, "Civic Engagement for Older Adults with Functional Limitations: Piloting an Intervention for Adult Day Health Participants," *Gerontologist*, Vol. 50, No. 5, 2010, pp. 694–701

Danso, K., "Immigrant Health Disparities: Does Neighborliness Improve Health?" *Journal of Sociology and Social Welfare*, Vol. 44, No. 3, 2017, pp. 75–94.

Davidson, William B., and Patrick R. Cotter, "The Relationship Between Sense of Community and Subjective Well-Being: A First Look," *Journal of Community Psychology*, Vol. 19, No. 3, 1991, pp. 246–253.

Den Broeder, Lea, Jeroean Devilee, Hans Van Oers, and A. Jantine Schuit, "Citizen Science for Public Health," *Health Promotion International*, Vol. 33, No. 3, June 2018. As of August 1, 2019: https://academic.oup.com/heapro/article/33/3/505/2623361

Denny, Kevin J., and Orla M. Doyle, "'. . .Take up Thy Bed, and Vote:' Measuring the Relationship Between Voting Behaviour and Indicators of Health," *European Journal of Public Health*, Vol. 17, No. 4, 2007, pp. 400–401.

Ding, N., H. L. Berry, and L. V. O'Brien, "One-Year Reciprocal Relationship Between Community Participation and Mental Wellbeing in Australia: A Panel Analysis," *Social Science and Medicine*, Vol. 128, 2015, pp. 246–254.

Downs, Anthony, "An Economic Theory of Democracy," in Ricardo Blaug and John Schwarzmantel, eds., *Democracy: A Reader*, New York: Columbia University Press, 1957.

Duke, N. N., C. L. Skay, S. L. Pettingell, and I. W. Borowsky, "From Adolescent Connections to Social Capital: Predictors of Civic Engagement in Young Adulthood," *Journal of Adolescent Health*, Vol. 44, No. 2, 2009, pp. 161–168.

Emerson, E., C. Hatton, J. Robertson, and S. Baines, "Perceptions of Neighbourhood Quality, Social and Civic Participation and the Self-Rated Health of British Adults with Intellectual Disability: Cross-Sectional Study," *BMC Public Health*, Vol. 14, No. 1, 2014.

Fang, S., N. L. Galambos, M. D. Johnson, and H. J. Krahn, "Happiness Is the Way: Paths to Civic Engagement Between Young Adulthood and Midlife," *International Journal of Behavioral Development*, Vol. 42, No. 4, 2018, pp. 425–433.

Finlay, A. K., and C. Flanagan, "Adolescents' Civic Engagement and Alcohol Use: Longitudinal Evidence for Patterns of Engagement and Use in the Adult Lives of a British Cohort," *Journal of Adolescence*, Vol. 36, No. 3, 2013, pp. 435–446.

Gerber, Alan S., Donald P. Green, and Christopher W. Larimer, "Social Pressure and Voter Turnout: Evidence from a Large-Scale Field Experiment," *American Political Science Review*, Vol. 102, No. 1, 2008, pp. 33–48.

Goetzel, Ron Z., Kevin Hawkins, Ronald J. Ozminkowski, and Shaohung Wang, "The Health and Productivity Cost Burden of the "Top 10" Physical and Mental Health Conditions Affecting Six Large U.S. Employers in 1999," *Journal of Occupational and Environmental Medicine*, Vol. 45, No. 1, 2003, pp. 5–14.

Gold, R., B. Kennedy, F. Connell, and I. Kawachi, "Teen Births, Income Inequality, and Social Capital: Developing an Understanding of the Causal Pathway," *Health and Place*, Vol. 8, No. 2, 2002, pp. 77–83.

Gollust, Sarah E., and Wendy M. Rahn, "The Bodies Politic: Chronic Health Conditions and Voter Turnout in the 2008 Election," *Journal of Health Politics, Policy and Law*, Vol. 40, No. 6, 2015, pp. 1115–1155.

Goth, U. S., and E. Småland, "The Role of Civic Engagement for Men's Health and Well-Being in Norway—A Contribution to Public Health," *International Journal of Environmental Research and Public Health*, Vol. 11, No. 6, 2014, pp. 6375–6387.

Grav, S., U. Romild, O. Hellzèn, and E. Stordal, "Association of Personality, Neighbourhood, and Civic Participation with the Level of Perceived Social Support: The HUNT Study, A Cross-Sectional Survey," *Scandinavian Journal of Public Health*, Vol. 41, No. 6, 2013, pp. 579–586.

Habibov, N., and R. Weaver, "Endogenous Social Capital and Self-Rated Health: Results from Canada's General Social Survey," *Health Sociology Review*, Vol. 23, No. 3, 2014, pp. 219–231.

Health Behaviour in School-Aged Survey, homepage, undated. As of July 31, 2019: http://www.hbsc.org

Highton, Benjamin, "Voter Identification Laws and Turnout in the United States," *Annual Review of Political Science*, Vol. 20, 2017, pp. 149–167.

Hobbs, William R., Nicholas A. Christakis, and James H. Fowler, "Widowhood Effects in Voter Participation," *American Journal of Political Science*, Vol. 58, No. 1, 2014, pp. 1–16.

Huckfeldt, Robert, and John Sprague, "Political Parties and Electoral Mobilization: Political Structure, Social Structure, and the Party Canvass," *American Political Science Review*, Vol. 86, No. 1, 1992, pp. 70–86.

Hyyppä, M. T., and J. Mäki, "Individual-Level Relationships Between Social Capital and Self-Rated Health in a Bilingual Community," *Preventive Medicine*, Vol. 32, No. 2, 2001, pp. 148–155.

Inglehart, Ronald, and Pippa Norris, *Rising Tide: Gender Equality and Cultural Change Around the World*, Cambridge, UK: Cambridge University Press, 2003.

Jennings, M. Kent, and Richard G. Niemi, *Generations and Politics: A Panel Study of Young Adults and Their Parents*, Vol. 68, Princeton, N. J.: Princeton University Press, 2014.

Kelleher, C., A. Timoney, S. Friel, and D. McKeown, "Indicators of Deprivation, Voting Patterns, and Health Status at Area Level in the Republic of Ireland," *Journal of Epidemiology and Community Health*, Vol. 56, No. 1, 2002.

Kelly, B. D., "Voting and Mental Illness: The Silent Constituency," *Irish Journal of Psychological Medicine*, Vol. 31, No. 4, 2014, pp. 225–227.

Kelly, B. D., and M. Nash, "Voter Participation Among People Attending Mental Health Services in Ireland," *Irish Journal of Medical Science*, October 2018.

Leedahl, S. N., A. M. Sellon, and N. Gallopyn, "Factors Predicting Civic Engagement among Older Adult Nursing Home Residents," *Activities, Adaptation and Aging*, Vol. 41, No. 3, 2017, pp. 197–219.

Leighley, Jan E., and Arnold Vedlitz, "Race, Ethnicity, and Political Participation: Competing Models and Contrasting Explanations," *Journal of Politics*, Vol. 61, No. 4, 1999, pp. 1092–1114.

Lenzi, M., A. Vieno, D. D. Perkins, M. Santinello, F. J. Elgar, A. Morgan, and S. Mazzardis, "Family Affluence, School and Neighborhood Contexts and Adolescents' Civic Engagement: A Cross-National Study," *American Journal of Community Psychology*, Vol. 50, No. 1–2, 2012, pp. 197–210.

Lindström, M., "Social Capital, Political Trust and Daily Smoking and Smoking Cessation: A Population-Based Study in Southern Sweden," *Public Health*, Vol. 123, No. 7, 2009, pp. 496–501. As of July 19, 2019: https://www.sciencedirect.com/science/article/abs/pii/S003335060900167X

Lochner, K. A., I. Kawachi, R. T. Brennan, and S. L. Buka, "Social Capital and Neighborhood Mortality Rates in Chicago," *Social Science and Medicine*, Vol. 56, No. 8, 2003, pp. 1797–1805.

Lubell, Mark, Sammy Zahran, and Arnold Vedlitz, "Collective Action and Citizen Responses to Global Warming," *Political Behavior*, Vol. 29, No. 3, 2007, pp. 391–413.

MacPhee, D., E. Forlenza, K. Christensen, and S. Prendergast, "Promotion of Civic Engagement with the Family Leadership Training Institute," *American Journal of Community Psychology*, Vol. 60, No. 3–4, 2017, pp. 568–583.

Mactaggart, F., L. McDermott, A. Tynan, and C. A. Gericke, "Exploring the Determinants of Health and Wellbeing in Communities Living in Proximity to Coal Seam Gas Developments in Regional Queensland," *BMC Public Health*, Vol. 18, No. 1, 2017.

Mahatmya, D., and B. J. Lohman, "Predictors and Pathways to Civic Involvement in Emerging Adulthood: Neighborhood, Family, and School Influences," *Journal of Youth and Adolescence*, Vol. 41, No. 9, 2012, pp. 1168–1183.

Manganelli, S., F. Lucidi, and F. Alivernini, "Italian Adolescents' Civic Engagement and Open Classroom Climate: The Mediating Role of Self-Efficacy," *Journal of Applied Developmental Psychology*, Vol. 41, 2015, pp. 8–18.

Marquez, B., P. Gonzalez, L. Gallo, and M. Ji, "Latino Civic Group Participation, Social Networks, and Physical Activity," *American Journal of Health Behavior*, Vol. 40, No. 4, 2016, pp. 437–445.

Mattila, Mikko, Peter Söderlund, Hanna Wass, and Lauri Rapeli, "Healthy Voting: The Effect of Self-Reported Health on Turnout in 30 Countries," *Electoral Studies*, Vol. 32, No. 4, 2013, pp. 886–891.

Mattila, Mikko, Hanna Wass, Hannu Lahtinen, and Pekka Martikainen, "Sick Leave from Work and the Voting Booth? A Register-Based Study on Health and Turnout," *Acta Politica*, Vol. 53, No. 3, 2018, pp. 429–447.

McClurg, Scott D., "Social Networks and Political Participation: The Role of Social Interaction in Explaining Political Participation," *Political Research Quarterly*, Vol. 56, No. 4, 2003, pp. 449–464.

Merzel, Cheryl, and Joanna D'Afflitti, "Reconsidering Community-Based Health Promotion: Promise, Performance, and Potential," *American Journal of Public Health*, Vol. 93, No. 4, 2003, pp. 557–574.

Mino, M., S. Deren, S. Y. Kang, and H. Guarino, "Associations Between Political/Civic Participation and HIV Drug Injection Risk," *American Journal of Drug and Alcohol Abuse*, Vol. 37, No. 6, 2011, pp. 520–524.

Navarro, Vicente, and Leiyu Shi, "The Political Context of Social Inequalities and Health," *International Journal of Health Services*, Vol. 31, No. 1, 2001, pp. 1–21.

Ojeda, Christopher, "Depression and Political Participation," *Social Science Quarterly*, Vol. 96, No. 5, 2015, pp. 1226–1243.

Ojeda, Christopher, and Julianna Pacheco, "Health and Voting in Young Adulthood," *British Journal of Political Science*, Vol. 49, No. 3, 2017, pp. 1–24.

Ott, B. R., W. C. Heindel, and G. D. Papandonatos, "A Survey of Voter Participation by Cognitively Impaired Elderly Patients," *Neurology*, Vol. 60, No. 9, 2003, pp. 1546–1548.

Petrou, S., and E. Kupek, "Social Capital and Its Relationship with Measures of Health Status: Evidence from the Health Survey for England 2003," *Health Economics*, Vol. 17, No. 1, 2008, pp. 127–143.

Pillemer, K., T. E. Fuller-Rowell, M. C. Reid, and N. M. Wells, "Environmental Volunteering and Health Outcomes over a 20-Year Period," *Gerontologist*, Vol. 50, No. 5, 2010, pp. 594–602.

Plough, A. L., "Building a Culture of Health: A Critical Role for Public Health Services and Systems Research," American Public Health Association, Washington, D.C., 2015.

Poortinga, W., "Social Capital: An Individual or Collective Resource for Health?" *Social Science and Medicine*, Vol. 62, No. 2, 2006, pp. 292–302.

Positive Psychology Center, "Psychological Well-Being Scales," webpage, undated. As of July 20, 2019:
https://ppc.sas.upenn.edu/resources/questionnaires-researchers/psychological-well-being-scales

Ramlagan, S., K. Peltzer, and N. Phaswana-Mafuya, "Social Capital and Health Among Older Adults in South Africa," *BMC Geriatrics*, Vol. 13, No. 1, 2013.

Ransome, Y., S. Galea, R. Pabayo, I. Kawachi, S. Braunstein, and D. Nash, "Social Capital Is Associated with Late HIV Diagnosis: An Ecological Analysis," *Journal of Acquired Immune Deficiency Syndromes*, Vol. 73, No. 2, 2016, pp. 213–221.

Republican National Committee, "2008 Republican Platform," St. Paul, Minn., 2008. As of May 17, 2013:
www.gop.com

———, "2012 Republican Platform—We Believe in America," Tampa, Fla., 2012. As of May 17, 2013:
www.gop.com

Robert Wood Johnson Foundation, "Civic Engagement," webpage, undated. As of July 31, 2019:
https://www.rwjf.org/en/cultureofhealth/taking-action/making-health-a-shared-value/civic-engagement.html

Schlozman, K. L., S. Verba, and H. E. Brady, *The Unheavenly Chorus: Unequal Political Voice and the Broken Promise of American Democracy*, Princeton, N.J.: Princeton University Press, 2012.

Schur, Lisa, Todd Shields, Douglas Kruse, and Kay Schriner, "Enabling Democracy: Disability and Voter Turnout," *Political Research Quarterly*, Vol. 55, No. 1, 2002, pp. 167–190.

Serrat, R., F. Villar, M. F. Giuliani, and J. J. Zacarés, "Older People's Participation in Political Organizations: The Role of Generativity and Its Impact on Well-Being," *Educational Gerontology*, Vol. 43, No. 3, 2017, pp. 128–138.

Shin, M. E., and W. J. McCarthy, "The Association Between County Political Inclination and Obesity: Results from the 2012 Presidential Election in the United States," *Preventive Medicine*, Vol. 57, No. 5, 2013, pp. 721–724.

Siegal, Gil, Neomi Siegal, and Richard J. Bonnie, "An Account of Collective Actions in Public Health," *American Journal of Public Health*, Vol. 99, No. 9, 2009, pp. 1583–1587.

Söderlund, Peter, and Lauri Rapeli, "In Sickness and in Health: Personal Health and Political Participation in the Nordic Countries," *Politics and the Life Sciences*, Vol. 34, No. 1, 2015, pp. 28–43.

Subica, A. M., C. T. Grills, S. Villanueva, and J. A. Douglas, "Community Organizing for Healthier Communities: Environmental and Policy Outcomes of a National Initiative," *American Journal of Preventive Medicine*, Vol. 51, No. 6, 2016, pp. 916–925.

Sund, Reijo, Hannu Lahtinen, Hanna Wass, Mikko Mattila, and Pekka Martikainen, "How Voter Turnout Varies Between Different Chronic Conditions? A Population-Based Register Study," *Journal of Epidemiology and Community Health*, Vol. 71, No. 5, 2016, pp. 475–479.

Taylor, L. K., "Impact of Political Violence, Social Trust, and Depression on Civic Participation in Colombia," *Peace and Conflict*, Vol. 22, No. 2, 2016, pp. 145–152.

Tomita, A., and J. K. Burns, "A Multilevel Analysis of Association Between Neighborhood Social Capital and Depression: Evidence from the First South African National Income Dynamics Study," *Journal of Affective Disorders*, Vol. 144, No. 1–2, 2013, pp. 101–105.

Urbatsch, R., "Influenza and Voter Turnout," *Scandinavian Political Studies*, Vol. 40, No. 1, 2017, pp. 107–119.

Van Groezen, B., R. Jadoenandansing, and G. Pasini, "Social Capital and Health Across European Countries," *Applied Economics Letters*, Vol. 18, No. 12, 2011, pp. 1167–1170.

Van Woerden, H. C., W. Poortinga, K. Bronstering, A. Garrib, and A. Hegazi, "The Relationship of Different Sources of Social Support and Civic Participation with Self-Rated Health," *Journal of Public Mental Health*, Vol. 10, No. 3, 2011, pp. 126–139.

Varma, V. R., M. C. Carlson, J. M. Parisi, E. K. Tanner, S. McGill, L. P. Fried, L. H. Song, and T. L. Gruenewald, "Experience Corps Baltimore: Exploring the Stressors and Rewards of High-Intensity Civic Engagement," *Gerontologist*, Vol. 55, No. 6, 2015, pp. 1038–1049.

Veenstra, G., "Social Capital, SES and Health: An Individual-Level Analysis," *Social Science and Medicine*, Vol. 50, No. 5, 2000, pp. 619–629.

———, "Social Capital and Health (Plus Wealth, Income Inequality and Regional Health Governance)," *Social Science and Medicine*, Vol. 54, No. 6, 2002, pp. 849–868.

Verba, Sidney, and Norman H. Nie, *Participation in America: Social Equality and Political Democracy*, New York: Harper & Row, 1972.

Wagenaar, A. C., D. M. Murray, J. P. Gehan, M. Wolfson, J. L. Forster, T. L. Toomey, C. L. Perry, and R. Jones-Webb, "Communities Mobilizing for Change on Alcohol: Outcomes from a Randomized Community Trial," *Journal of Studies on Alcohol*, Vol. 61, No. 1, 2000, pp. 85–94. As of August 1, 2019: https://www.jsad.com/doi/abs/10.15288/jsa.2000.61.85

Wass, H., M. Mattila, L. Rapeli, and P. Söderlund, "Voting While Ailing? The Effect of Voter Facilitation Instruments on Health-Related Differences in Turnout," *Journal of Elections, Public Opinion and Parties*, Vol. 27, No. 4, 2017, pp. 503–522.

Wolfinger, Nicholas H., and Raymond E. Wolfinger, "Family Structure and Voter Turnout," *Social Forces*, Vol. 86, No. 4, 2008, pp. 1513–1528.

Wolstenholme, Eric F., "Towards the Definition and Use of a Core Set of Archetypal Structures in System Dynamics," *System Dynamics Review*, Vol. 19, No. 1, 2003, pp. 7–26.

Wray-Lake, Laura, Jennifer Shubert, Lin Lin, and Lisa R. Starr, "Examining Associations Between Civic Engagement and Depressive Symptoms from Adolescence to Young Adulthood in a National U.S. Sample," *Applied Developmental Science*, Vol. 23, No. 2, June 30, 2017, pp. 1–13.

Wu, Q., and J. C. Chow, "Social Service Utilization, Sense of Community, Family Functioning and the Mental Health of New Immigrant Women in Hong Kong," *International Journal of Environmental Research and Public Health*, Vol. 10, No. 5, April 29, 2013, pp. 1735–1746. As of August 1, 2019: http://www.ncbi.nlm.nih.gov/pubmed/23629592

Zhu, L., "Healing Alone? Social Capital, Racial Diversity and Health Care Inequality in the American States," *American Politics Research*, Vol. 45, No. 6, 2017, pp. 1059–1087.

Ziegenfuss, J. K., M. Davern, and L. A. Blewett, "Access to Health Care and Voting Behavior in the United States," *Journal of Health Care for the Poor and Underserved*, Vol. 19, No. 3, August 2008, pp. 731–742.

Ziersch, A. M., F. Baum, I. G. N. Darmawan, A. M. Kavanagh, and R. J. Bentley, "Social Capital and Health in Rural and Urban Communities in South Australia," *Australian and New Zealand Journal of Public Health*, Vol. 33, No. 1, 2009, pp. 7–16.